Cranks
Light

To Digby and Noah, with love

Author's acknowledgements
In writing this book, I have had lots of help and support from many people.
In particular, I'd like to express my very heartfelt thanks to Gavin Heys,
managing director of Cranks; Yvonne Bishop for checking the nutritional
status of all the recipes; Sian Owen for help in recipe testing; Laura
Washburn and Maggie Ramsay at Weidenfeld & Nicolson; and to my
family and friends for their love, encouragement and assistance.

First published in Great Britain in 1998
by Weidenfeld & Nicolson

This paperback edition first published in 1999 by
Seven Dials, Illustrated Division
The Orion Publishing Group
Wellington House, 125 Strand
London, WC2R 0BB

A CIP catalogue record for this book is available from the British Library

ISBN 1 84188 018 3

Designed by Nigel Soper

Copy edited by Maggie Ramsay
Home economy by Debbie Miller, Maxine Clark, Louise Pickford
Styling by Penny Markham

Nadine Abensur

Cranks Light

100 Recipes for Health and Vitality

Photographs by Gus Filgate

Nutritional Consultant:
Suzannah Olivier

SEVEN DIALS

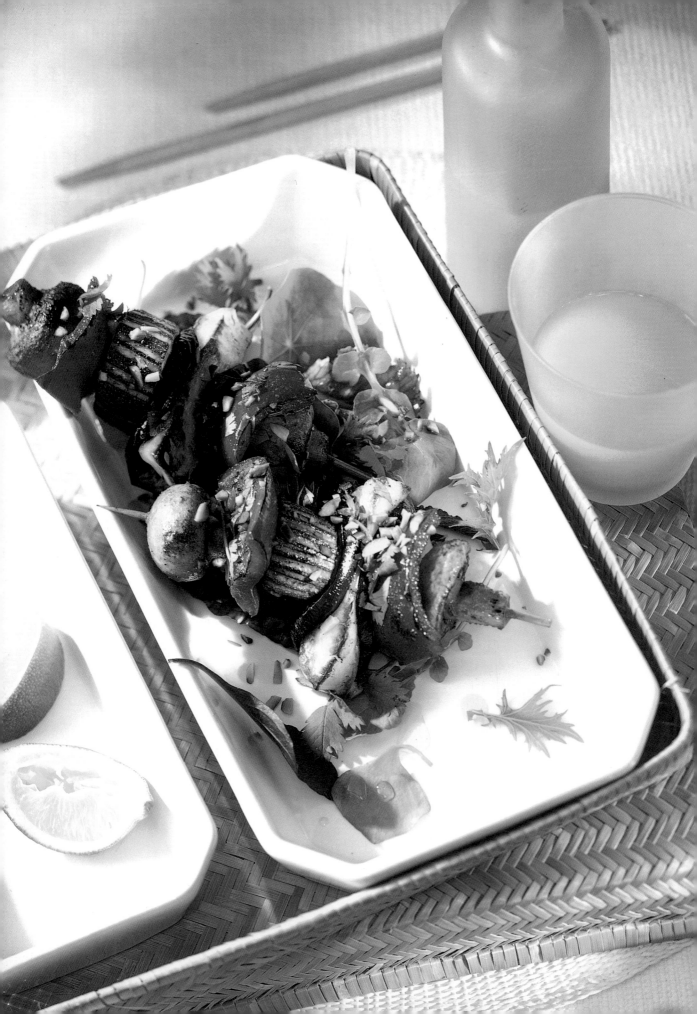

Contents

THE CRANKS VISION

Born in the sixties, Cranks restaurants were a direct response to growing consumer awareness of the benefits of a more natural and healthy diet. Our objective was to provide the best **quality** for our customers – food from Cranks was always fresh, prepared with care and filled with **natural goodness** making it a pleasure to eat.

Cranks is buzzing again In today's fast-moving world, the need for fresh healthy food has never been greater, and Cranks is still at the forefront. We live more pressurized, more crowded lives, in which stress levels are high. Time poverty has replaced material poverty as one of our greatest hardships, and the **temptation** to eat whatever is fast and easily to hand is stronger. The typical lunch hour is now just twenty minutes, reduced to a sandwich snatched at a desk, and preparation of the evening meal has been replaced by the **convenience** of microwaved ready meals.

What people need is food that **revitalizes** and **strengthens**. But what is on offer, passing under the banner of fast-food, can barely pass muster as **nourishment**. At least, not in the way we think of it at Cranks.

A Radical Transformation In the face of this tidal wave of junk food, and armed with the latest consensus thinking from dietary and nutritional science, Cranks has **radically** transformed itself to meet today's convenience eating needs. Our Vitality and Health Cafés offer what we call the **best food for vitality and health**. Delicious, healthy food that is good for you and makes you feel great – no trade-offs. We use only fresh and natural ingredients, avoiding additives and preservatives. There are no synthetic fat substitutes, no guar or xanthan gums, no emulsifiers, and none of the fillers that provide bulk without **nutrition** – these simply bring down manufacturing costs at the expense of the quality of the food.

From government research we all know that reducing fat, increasing fibre and eating more fruit and vegetables is **essential** for our long-term well-being. At Cranks we make this easier for our customers by doing the hard work for them. All Cranks products undergo strict nutritional **analysis**. We aim to offer food that is low in saturated fat, high in fibre and we rarely use sugar, except for desserts. If a recipe cannot be made with **natural**, fresh ingredients and meet our **criterion** of having less than 40% of its calories from fat, we simply don't make it.

Nutrition Today The definition of a healthy diet has changed dramatically over the last three or four decades. Not so long ago an egg and bacon breakfast, followed by a spaghetti Bolognese lunch and a meat supper with fried potatoes and custardy pudding would have seemed **normal**. Now it would be considered a recipe for heart disease and certain forms of cancer. What has changed is our understanding of the **role** of protein, fats and carbohydrate in the diet.

Fats Fat is increasingly seen as the main barrier to achieving a healthier diet for two key reasons. Firstly, fat is an intense source of calories, containing twice the number of calories, gram for gram, as carbohydrates or protein. The calories that we fail to **burn off** are stored by the body as fat. Secondly, a high intake of saturated fat (especially found in meat and butter) is associated with raised blood cholesterol levels and increased levels of heart disease.

Government guidelines suggest that no more than one-third of calories should come from fat, and many authorities say it should be **lower** still. The average person in Britain obtains 40% of calories from fat. Not all fat is bad fat. Polyunsaturated fats (found in plants, vegetables and oily fish) are thought to **decrease** cholesterol. Monounsaturated fats, such as olive oil, are believed to do the same, and this is why the Mediterranean diet has received so much attention. Fates must not be cut out altogether as they form a necessary part of our diet. They help to transport certain vitamins around the body, and are an **essential** component of all cell structures, nervous tissue and some hormones.

Protein The paradox of the Western diet is that it contains more than enough protein. The fact is that the body possesses the ability to manufacture most of its requirements from the store of amino acids (the "building blocks" of proteins) in the liver. Only about 40 g needs to come from the food we eat. No vegetarian or vegan need fear they are **lacking** in protein, especially as long as they eat a variety of grains (breakfast cereals, bread, pasta, rice, couscous), nuts and pulses (peas, beans and lentils). Since the average diet obtains much of its protein from fat-rich foods such as meat, eggs and dairy produce, the issue of **excess** fat is exacerbated by the over-consumption of protein-rich foods. This is not to diminish the crucial role of protein. It is essential for the health of all our body cells, as well as the hormones, enzymes and nerve chemicals that pass messages around our bodies.

Carbohydrates Our understanding of the role of carbohydrate has come a long way since the days when sugary and starchy foods were branded together as 'fuel food'. Today, a clear distinction is made between simple carbohydrates – basically the sugars, such as sucrose, fructose, glucose and honey – and complex carbohydrates: starchy foods that are low in fat and **packed** with vitamins, minerals and fibre. These include bread, pasta and other cereal products, as well as vegetables and fruit. Although fibre is not digested, it provides **valuable** bulk that enables our bodies to process food efficiently. Lack of fibre has been clearly linked with many types of cancer, heart disease, diabetes and bowel disease. Healthy eating guidelines recommend at least five daily portions of fruit and vegetables. For **optimum** nutrition and vitality, choose a mixture of different seasonal produce: green vegetables; red, orange and yellow fruit and vegetables such as peppers, carrots, melons and apricots; citrus fruits; root vegetables.

Nutritional Guidelines

The Department of Health's Dietary Reference Values for a healthy 20 to 40-year-old woman of average activity gives benchmark figures of 1,940 calories, which can include up to 71 g of fat (we tend to eat more than this) and 36 g of protein (we tend to eat enough). The recommended 18 g of dietary fibre represents a **staggering** 50% suggested increase in our current average consumption. Some authorities (such as the American Cancer Institute) recommend even more fibre – around 25–35g a day. To put these figures into **context**, a typical Cranks main course would provide 300–400 calories, 10–15 g of fat and 5–15 g of fibre; 25–35% of its calories come from fat.

A New Way of Eating

About half of the fat we eat comes from meat or dairy products, and the rest mainly from cakes, biscuits and fried foods, with some from cereal products and oily fish. Cutting down on the first category is the obvious place to start. By **enjoying** more of the very low fat foods such as fruit and vegetables, and foods that are high in carbohydrates, you will soon find that your **craving** for added sugar and fat-rich foods is diminished. Do not think of it as **deprivation** but rather as a new way of eating with quite as much variety as the old. It may take a while to break certain habits, but you should find that your liking for greasy foods will disappear as you not only enjoy the cleaner, fresher tastes of this kind of cooking but also start to feel new levels of **health** and **vitality**.

Today, a healthy day's menus might begin with a breakfast of fruit and wholemeal toast, muesli or other breakfast cereal. Lunch could be a sandwich **packed** with vegetables and salad leaves, a plate of three different salads, one of them grain-based, or a vegetable soup and a chunk of wholemeal bread. A supper of baked, roasted or stir-fried vegetables with brown rice, pasta or couscous might be followed by a fruit-based pudding with yoghurt.

A new approach to cooking This may sound easy on paper, but unless you are used to eating a healthy diet, it can be difficult to know where to start when so much of the food on offer blatantly does not meet this criteria. Cranks take the effort out of healthy eating by making it **enjoyable** and **accessible**, never forgetting that great recipes win "in the mouth".

The recipes in this book reflect **current thinking**. They show you how to reduce the fat in your diet, using new techniques that concentrate the food's flavour. The Western diet has typically been a fat-rich one, heavy on cholesterol-high dairy produce. By contrast the cooking of many parts of the East is much lower in fat. This is partly due to the lack of dairy produce and partly to regional cooking techniques that remain low in fat without sacrificing **taste**. This book uses these and develops others more akin to Western recipes.

You will be surprised at how easy it is to roast vegetables using substantially less oil than is traditional, simply by adding a little water or other liquid ingredients, which help to disperse the fat molecules. Also, because fat expands when it is heated, a little can go a long way. Alternatively, vegetables are partly blanched first and then roasted to a **crisp** and **golden** finish. You will find that blanching vegetables for a few seconds lessens their need for oil, which is often only added to achieve the desired browning and caramelization of the sugars. Slow cooking encourages the **release** of the vegetables' own juices. Non-stick pots and pans help, especially if they are heavy-bottomed.

I have seldom used steaming as a technique in the book, because **my aim** was to create recipes that are lower in fat than usual, not necessarily to create fat-free ones. But you couldn't go wrong with a plateful of lightly steamed vegetables served with any one of the many low fat dressings found in the Salads chapter.

Lower fat dairy products are used, but most recipes do away with them altogether. It is easy to fulfil high fibre recommendations because these recipes are based around vegetables, fruit and pulses.

In the restaurants, we look at each item individually to see that nothing derives more than 40% of its calories from fat (most are considerably lower but at the very least you can always know that you are doing better than the UK average). This ensures that your lunchtime needs are nutritionally **soundly** met. To be totally accurate in our nutritional analyses, we use standard measuring spoons: 1 tablespoon = 15 ml; 1 teaspoon = 5 ml. You may find the use of measuring spoons disconcerting, but it is an **effective** and **accurate** way of conveying information. Occasionally, when you are making the recipes at home, you might add a generous garnish of nuts, seeds, cheese or a drizzle of olive oil. This would nudge up the fat content – but we don't expect anyone to analyze every mouthful, and of course it's up to you to decide how **strictly** you need to control your fat intake, depending on your individual circumstances.

We would hate for people to become obsessive fat counters (in the way that many women became calorie counters in the seventies), but this book should help you begin to make healthy food choices. Don't forget that while some recipes have more fat than others, a whole day's menus based on the Cranks style of eating will, overall, provide a healthy, **balanced** diet. And by using plenty of fresh fruit and vegetables you will be doing your body a favour and end up feeling full of **vitality**.

Amid all this talk of health and nutrition, we must never forget that delicious food is our first priority. Nothing beats using **fresh** ingredients, good oils, herbs and spices, and condiments from around the world. Taste, above all, measures a recipe's success and I have paid particular attention to this. Sooner or later you will want to follow your own instincts: you may like your food more or less highly flavoured than I do; you may be **inspired** to change an ingredient here or there, or to create new recipes altogether – that is part of the **fun** of cooking.

SOUPS AND STARTERS

Nothing beats a fresh, **homemade soup** – its savoury aromas will stimulate the appetite. Lightly simmered vegetables can be blended to create a smooth and elegant soup with very little fat, or none at all, but they need to be well seasoned and garnished. Soups are also a great way of using whatever's to hand and are easily made in large quantities. They can form the base of a **sustaining** lunchtime meal, or can be served as a starter to a more traditional supper.

Three-course meals are an endangered species, but sitting down to a dinner with a **light** first course creates a sense of occasion and sets a leisurely pace, vital for the full enjoyment of any meal. Starters can be of quite **intense** flavour because the servings tend to be smaller, whether they are plated in advance – a great excuse for showing off – or shared out at the table.

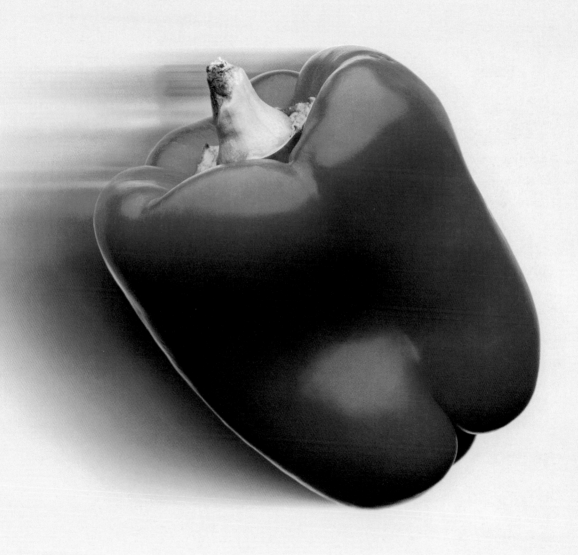

Mushroom consommé

SERVES 4

INGREDIENTS
1 teaspoon **olive oil**

250 g/9 oz assorted fresh **mushrooms**
  (chanterelles, shiitake, trompettes de mort,
  oyster mushrooms), tough stalks removed (use
  for stock), then sliced

1 tablespoon **tamari**

bunch of **chives**

VEGETABLE STOCK
2 **carrots**, cut into small chunks

1 **leek**, sliced

3 sticks of **celery**, chopped

25 g/1 oz dried **mushrooms**

50 g/2 oz **brown lentils**

5 **garlic cloves**, peeled

2 **spring onions**, chopped

8–9 **peppercorns**

the stalks from the fresh mushrooms

handful of fresh **coriander**

900 ml/1½ pints water

Nothing concentrates the flavours of mushrooms quite like garlic and tamari; the intensity is almost intoxicating.

METHOD
1. Put all the ingredients for the stock into a saucepan. Bring to the boil, then reduce the heat and simmer for 40 minutes. Pour through a sieve into a clean saucepan, squeezing through as much liquid as possible.
2. Heat the olive oil in a separate pan. Add the sliced mushrooms and tamari and sauté for 1–2 minutes, until just beginning to soften. Add a little water if necessary to prevent sticking. Add to the stock and return to the boil, then serve immediately, sprinkled with snipped chives.

NUTRITIONAL INFORMATION
one serving contains

CALORIES	106
TOTAL FAT	2.8 G
CARBOHYDRATES	13.2 G
TOTAL SUGAR	5.2 G
FIBRE	5.7 G
SODIUM	0.7 G

Roasted cherry tomato soup

SERVES 4

INGREDIENTS

1.5 kg/3 lb **cherry tomatoes**

1 tablespoon **olive oil**

sea salt and freshly ground black pepper

3 **garlic cloves**, peeled

small handful of fresh **basil** sprigs

4 tablespoons **yoghurt**

It may seem sacrilegious, not to say overly fussy, to take something as sweet and pretty as a ripe cherry tomato, then roast and blend it out of all recognition, but I've made many fresh tomato soups and none have come out quite as full of flavour as this one. I'm told that sieving food is one of my foibles, but it is essential for this soup, which should be as perfectly smooth as possible.

The roasted tomatoes (step 1) are also delicious on bruschetta, with spaghetti, rice or couscous.

METHOD

1. Heat the oven to 200°C/400°F/gas 6. Coat the tomatoes with the oil, salt and pepper. Place on a baking sheet and roast in the hot oven for 10–15 minutes, or until the skins are beginning to shrivel and blacken.

2. Tip the tomatoes into a blender or food processor and blend until smooth, then rub through a sieve into a saucepan.

3. Place over a low heat and add the whole garlic cloves and most of the basil. Simmer gently for 10–15 minutes, then remove the basil and garlic. Add up to 100 ml/3½ fl oz water to thin down the consistency, if preferred. Serve in soup plates, with a spoonful of yoghurt, a small sprig of basil and a sprinkling of coarsely ground black pepper.

NUTRITIONAL INFORMATION
one serving contains

CALORIES:	114
TOTAL FAT:	5.4 G
CARBOHYDRATES:	13 G
TOTAL SUGAR:	12.4 G
FIBRE:	3.9 G
SODIUM:	0.6 G

Jerusalem artichoke,
walnut and rocket soup

SERVES 4–5

INGREDIENTS

1 large red **onion**, cut into chunks

4 **garlic cloves**, peeled and left whole

700 g/1½ lb **Jerusalem artichokes**, peeled
   and cut into chunks

1.5 litres/2½ pints vegetable stock or water

85 g/3 oz **rocket**

25 g/1 oz **walnuts**, chopped

salt and pepper

1 teaspoon lemon juice (optional)

1 tablespoon walnut oil (optional)

French **bread** or wholemeal bread, to serve

These three strong, earthy flavours need to be carefully balanced. Pecan nuts or hazelnuts would make a sweeter alternative to the walnuts.

METHOD

1. Put the onion, garlic and artichokes in a large saucepan and add just over half the stock or water. Boil for about 20–25 minutes, until the artichokes are just tender.

2. Add the rest of the stock and three-quarters of the rocket and simmer for 1 minute, then add the walnuts and purée in a blender.

3. Season to taste, adding a little lemon juice if you think it needs it. Serve hot, garnished with the remaining rocket leaves, and drizzle on a little walnut oil (unless you want to control your fat intake more strictly). Serve with bread to make a nourishing lunch or supper.

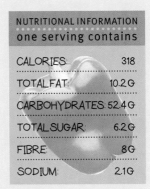

NUTRITIONAL INFORMATION
one serving contains

CALORIES:	318
TOTAL FAT:	10.2 G
CARBOHYDRATES:	52.4 G
TOTAL SUGAR:	6.2 G
FIBRE:	8 G
SODIUM:	2.1 G

Broad bean and cumin soup
with a sun-dried tomato and black olive concassé

SERVES 6

INGREDIENTS
3 **shallots**, finely chopped

1 teaspoon **olive oil**

2 teaspoons ground **cumin**

2 **garlic cloves**, finely sliced

good pinch of **bouillon powder**

1.2 litres/2 pints vegetable stock

pinch of **saffron** threads, soaked in
   3 tablespoons boiling water

1 kg/2¼ lb frozen **broad beans**

1 teaspoon **tamari**

salt and pepper

TO SERVE
6 pieces of **sun-dried tomatoes**
   (dried and ready-to-eat, not preserved in oil),
   finely chopped

12 **black olives**, finely diced

150 g/5 oz **yoghurt**

As an alternative topping, try this soup garnished with some finely sliced mushrooms, sautéed in a dash of olive oil and some tamari. Even a little browned garlic, something I usually avoid, is great and gives the soup a kick.

Broad beans are high in protein and a good source of calcium and iron as well as vitamins A, B1 and B2. For a fascinating account of their history and the mythology surrounding them, read Colin Spencer's Vegetable Book.

METHOD
1. Gently fry the shallots in the olive oil until they are soft and translucent. Add the cumin, garlic, bouillon powder and a little stock and simmer for a few minutes.
2. Add the saffron and its soaking liquid, the broad beans and remaining stock, return to the boil and simmer for 10 minutes.
3. Add the tamari, then pour into a blender and purée until smooth. Season to taste with salt and pepper. Reheat gently and serve in individual bowls, garnished with sun-dried tomatoes, olives and a spoonful of yoghurt.

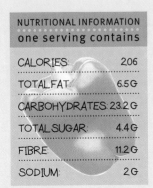

NUTRITIONAL INFORMATION one serving contains	
CALORIES:	206
TOTAL FAT:	6.5 G
CARBOHYDRATES:	23.2 G
TOTAL SUGAR:	4.4 G
FIBRE:	11.2 G
SODIUM:	2 G

Japanese broth

SERVES 4

INGREDIENTS

125 g/4 oz **tofu**, cut into thin strips

2 tablespoons **tamari**

1 **carrot**

2 tablespoons **rice vinegar**

900 ml/1½ pints vegetable stock

100 g/3½ oz **baby corn**, cut in half lengthways

100 g/3½ oz **mangetout**, topped and tailed, cut diagonally

1 bunch of **spring onions**, cut diagonally

175 g/6 oz **shiitake mushrooms**, thickly sliced

2 cm/¾ inch piece of fresh **ginger**, finely grated

2 tablespoons **ume su** (pickled plum vinegar)

1 tablespoon **sherry**

dash of **Tabasco** sauce

2 teaspoons **seaweed** (nori) flakes

small handful of fresh **coriander**

Try this light, low-calorie soup before a stir-fry or as part of an entire Japanese meal, including sushi (page 32), filled wontons (page 82), pickled vegetable salad (page 74) and a simple array of sliced exotic fruit or a bowl of lychees to follow.

If you like, you could add a spoonful of miso (fermented soybean paste) to the soup. Miso is full of B vitamins and is considered to be an antidote to the over-rich foods we tend to consume.

METHOD

1. Marinate the tofu strips in the tamari for at least 2 hours. Cut five grooves along the length of the carrot, then cut it into thin, flower-shaped slices, cover with the rice vinegar and leave for about 2 hours.

2. Bring the vegetable stock to the boil and add the corn, mangetout, spring onions and mushrooms. Bring back to the boil and simmer for about 3 minutes.

3. Squeeze in the juice from the ginger, then stir in the ume su, sherry, Tabasco and seaweed flakes. Add the tofu and tamari, garnish with the carrot flowers and coriander and serve at once.

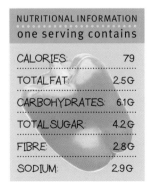

NUTRITIONAL INFORMATION one serving contains	
CALORIES	79
TOTAL FAT	2.5 G
CARBOHYDRATES	6.1 G
TOTAL SUGAR	4.2 G
FIBRE	2.8 G
SODIUM	2.9 G

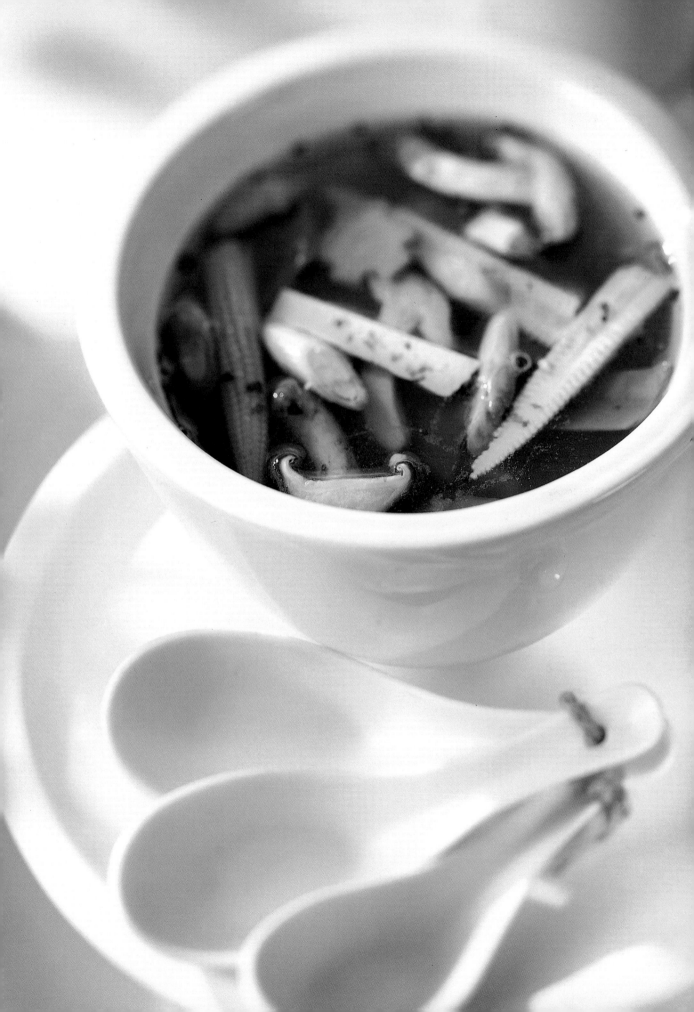

Light lentil soup
with herb 'quenelles'

SERVES 6

INGREDIENTS
250 g/9 oz **lentils**

3 **garlic cloves**, peeled

1 small **red onion**, sliced

3 big pieces of dried **porcini mushrooms**

good pinch of **saffron** threads, added to
500 ml/16 fl oz hot water

1 teaspoon ground **cumin**

1 teaspoon **paprika**

1 litre/1¾ pints vegetable stock

1 teaspoon sun-dried **tomato purée**

1 tablespoon **tamari**

dash of **balsamic vinegar**

dash of **Tabasco** sauce

salt and pepper

TO GARNISH
small bunch of **parsley**

small bunch of **coriander**

1 tablespoon **olive oil**

small piece of **fresh chilli**, finely chopped

Lentils usually mean a thick, hearty soup but I wanted to go against expectation; the result turned out to be delicious and no less earthy in its flavours. Lentils are a good source of protein.

METHOD
1. Put the lentils into a large saucepan, together with the garlic, onion, dried mushrooms, saffron liquid, cumin and paprika. Add the stock and bring to the boil, then reduce the heat and simmer for about 20 minutes.
2. Add 700 ml/1¼ pints of water and simmer for about 20 minutes more, or until the lentils are tender.
3. Blend, then rub through a sieve. Stir in the tomato purée, tamari, vinegar and Tabasco. Taste and adjust the seasoning if necessary.
4. For the garnish, finely chop the parsley and coriander and mix with the olive oil and chopped chilli. Shape into small quenelles and place in the centre of each bowl of soup.

NUTRITIONAL INFORMATION
one serving contains

CALORIES:	180
TOTAL FAT:	3.9 G
CARBOHYDRATES:	27.4 G
TOTAL SUGAR:	2.2 G
FIBRE:	2.5 G
SODIUM:	0.6 G

Mixed vegetable soup

SERVES 6

INGREDIENTS

2 tablespoons **olive oil**

1 small **onion**, diced

2 small **potatoes**, diced

2 sticks of **celery**, sliced

1 large **carrot**, cut into chunks

1 **leek**, finely sliced

2 **garlic cloves**, peeled

1 **small courgette**, cut into 1 cm/½ inch thick
  slices

¼ medium **cauliflower**, cut into florets

¼ medium **white cabbage**, cut into small
  chunks

400 g/14 oz **pumpkin**, peeled and cut into small
  chunks

2 **bay leaves**

1 litre/1¾ pints vegetable stock or water

1 teaspoon **bouillon powder**

handful of **basil** sprigs

1 tablespoon **tamari**

salt and pepper

An everyday, warming, reassuring refuge after a long day's work. Nothing makes me feel like I've come home quite like a bowl of this soup. Some people prefer chunky soups, others like them velvety smooth. I am definitely of the latter category. Even this soup seems sophisticated when smooth, served with a spoonful of bio yoghurt in the middle, a few twists of the pepper mill and some finely snipped chives.

METHOD

1. Heat the oil in a large saucepan, add the onion and fry until translucent. Add the remaining vegetables and the bay leaves and just enough stock or water to cover. Bring to the boil, stirring regularly for about 10 minutes.

2. Add the remaining stock or water and the bouillon powder and boil for abut 20 minutes, adding most of the basil sprigs for the last 10 minutes.

3. Remove the basil and bay leaves, add the tamari and blend until very smooth. Season to taste and serve hot, garnished with cracked black pepper and small sprigs of basil.

NUTRITIONAL INFORMATION
one serving contains

CALORIES	137
TOTAL FAT	6.1 G
CARBOHYDRATES	17 G
TOTAL SUGAR	7.5 G
FIBRE	4.3 G
SODIUM	1 G

Green spring soup

SERVES 6

INGREDIENTS

½ teaspoon **olive oil**

3 **spring onions** (white parts), finely sliced

100 g/3½ oz canned **flageolet beans**, drained

1.5 litres/2½ pints boiling vegetable stock

250 g/9 oz baby **broad beans**, blanched,
  refreshed and skinned

250 g/9 oz **petit pois**

3 **garlic cloves**, finely sliced

125 g/4 oz young **asparagus** spears

1 tablespoon chopped fresh **chives**

1 tablespoon finely chopped **sorrel**

juice of ½ lemon

2–3 teaspoons **wholegrain mustard**

salt and pepper

This makes the most of fresh broad beans, fresh peas and fresh asparagus in their all-too-short season, which I know comes a little later than spring – the name is somewhat poetic. Green vegetables are high in iron.

METHOD

1. Heat the olive oil and briefly sauté the spring onions. Add the flageolet beans and hot stock and simmer for 5 minutes. Add the broad beans, peas and garlic and simmer for 2–3 minutes.

2. Cut off the tips of the asparagus and finely slice the stems. Add the asparagus to the soup, together with the chives and sorrel, and simmer for a further 3–4 minutes.

3. Just before serving, squeeze in some lemon juice and stir in the mustard, and salt and pepper to taste. Serve at once: don't allow the soup to stand after you have added the lemon juice or the acid will turn the green vegetables brown.

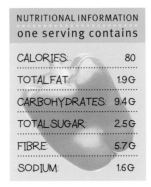

NUTRITIONAL INFORMATION
one serving contains

CALORIES	80
TOTAL FAT	1.9 G
CARBOHYDRATES	9.4 G
TOTAL SUGAR	2.5 G
FIBRE	5.7 G
SODIUM	1.6 G

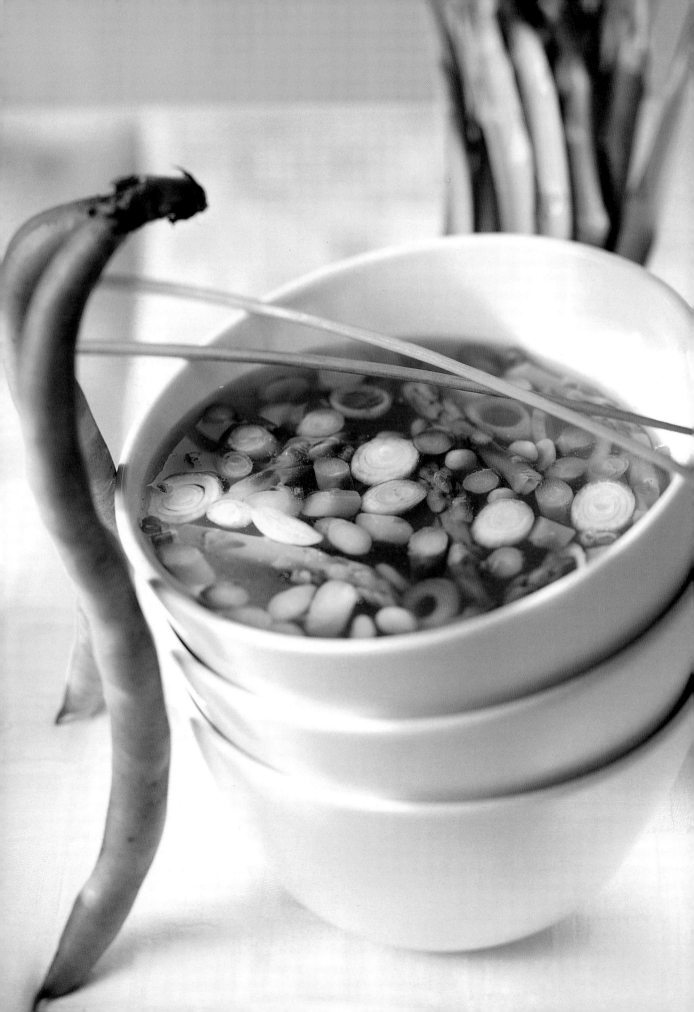

Layered focaccia
with red peppers and avocados

SERVES 6

INGREDIENTS
2 **red peppers**

1 round **tomato focaccia**

1 large **avocado**

25 g/1 oz **rocket**

6 **pistachio nuts**, roughly chopped (optional)

FIVE-HERB DRESSING
3 tablespoons chopped fresh **basil**

1½ tablespoons chopped fresh **sorrel**

3 tablespoons chopped fresh **coriander**

3 tablespoons chopped fresh **chives**

1 tablespoon chopped fresh **parsley**

1 **garlic clove**, crushed

5 tablespoons **yoghurt**

5 tablespoons **fromage frais**

dash of **Tabasco** sauce

sea salt and freshly ground black pepper

There must be six of you to eat this so that you can appreciate it in all its tricoloured, catherine-wheeled glory. The pistachio nuts are a pretty addition, but it's up to you to decide whether you can afford the fat, since they take the percentage of calories from fat slightly over the 40% mark. Reserve the top layer of bread to make yourself a sandwich the next day.

METHOD
1. Preheat the oven to 180°C/350°F/gas 4. Preheat the grill. Grill the red peppers until the skin is blackened all over. Leave to cool slightly, then remove all the skin and cut the peppers into narrow strips.
2. Mix together all the ingredients for the dressing, adding 1 tablespoon water, with Tabasco, salt and pepper to taste.
3. Warm the focaccia through in the oven for about 8–10 minutes, then leave to cool slightly. Using a bread knife, slice the bread horizontally into three large rounds.
4. Cut the avocado in half, remove the stone and skin, and slice thinly.
5. Put the bottom layer of bread on a board, then arrange half the pepper and avocado on top in a pinwheel pattern. Cover with the second layer of bread and repeat the layer of pepper and avocado. Scatter the rocket around the focaccia, spoon on the dressing and scatter over the pistachios, if using. To serve, cut the focaccia into six slices, like a cake.

NUTRITIONAL INFORMATION
one serving contains

CALORIES:	346
TOTAL FAT:	15.8 G
CARBOHYDRATES:	43.6 G
TOTAL SUGAR:	8.4 G
FIBRE:	4 G
SODIUM:	1.2 G

Avocado mousse
with beef tomatoes

SERVES 6

INGREDIENTS

1 large ripe **avocado**

1 **garlic clove**, crushed

sea salt and freshly ground black pepper

¼ **red onion**, finely diced

3 large **beef tomatoes**

6 slices of **French bread**, cut diagonally,
   toasted and left until cold

6 small **basil** sprigs

125 g/4 oz salad leaves

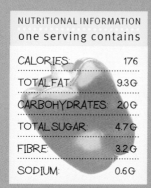

NUTRITIONAL INFORMATION
one serving contains

CALORIES:	176
TOTAL FAT:	9.3 G
CARBOHYDRATES:	20 G
TOTAL SUGAR:	4.7 G
FIBRE:	3.2 G
SODIUM:	0.6 G

I always use Hass avocados when possible: their flesh is creamier and more 'buttery' than other varieties. In this elegant starter, the sharpness of the tomato eases the richness and the whole thing is as delicate a starter as any. Here, the avocado nudges the percentage of calories from fat a little over the recommended 40%, but since it is clearly a light first course, the rest of the meal is sure to balance out nutritionally. You must prepare avocado very much at the last minute – lemon juice will only keep it from going black for a short time. Fresh sea salt and black pepper – the other two essentials for avocado – appear in the dressing.

METHOD

1. Put the avocado, garlic, salt, pepper and 2 tablespoons water into a blender or food processor and blend to a coarse purée. Mix in the finely diced onion. Set aside 1 tablespoon of the avocado mousse.

2. Cut each tomato into six slices, discarding a thin slice from each end. Scrape the tomato seeds into a sieve over a bowl to catch the juice.

3. Place a slice of toasted French bread on each plate. On top of this, place a slice of tomato, a thin layer of avocado mousse, another slice of tomato and layer of avocado, and finish with a slice of tomato. Top with a small sprig of basil and arrange the salad leaves around the plate.

4. Mix the reserved avocado mousse with the tomato juice and drizzle over the salad leaves. Serve at once.

Leeks with five-herb dressing

SERVES 4

INGREDIENTS

8 young **leeks**, about 3 cm/1 inch diameter,
  trimmed to remove any tough green parts, then
  cut into 4–5 cm/1½–2 inch lengths
chopped **chives**
1 **lime**, cut into 4 wedges
a few **black olives** (optional)

FIVE-HERB DRESSING

3 tablespoons chopped fresh **basil**
1½ tablespoons chopped fresh **sorrel**
3 tablespoons chopped fresh **coriander**
3 tablespoons chopped fresh **chives**
1 tablespoon chopped fresh **parsley**
150 g/5 oz **yoghurt**
1 **garlic clove**, crushed
dash of **Tabasco** sauce
sea salt and freshly ground black pepper

Occasionally you'll find baby leeks, thin as pencils – this fabulously fresh-tasting dressing is the perfect way to serve them. It's also packed with vitamins and minerals – among others, it's a good source of folic acid.

METHOD

1. Mix together all the ingredients for the dressing, adding 1 tablespoon water, with Tabasco, salt and pepper to taste. Set aside.
2. Blanch the leeks in boiling salted water for 3–4 minutes, then drain and dry on kitchen paper.
3. Divide the leeks between four serving plates, piling them in a pyramid shape. Pour the dressing over the top and sprinkle with chives. Serve a wedge of lime on the side. If you like, scatter a few black olives around the plates. Serve warm.

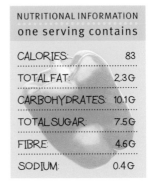

NUTRITIONAL INFORMATION
one serving contains

CALORIES:	83
TOTAL FAT:	2.3 G
CARBOHYDRATES:	10.1 G
TOTAL SUGAR:	7.5 G
FIBRE:	4.6 G
SODIUM:	0.4 G

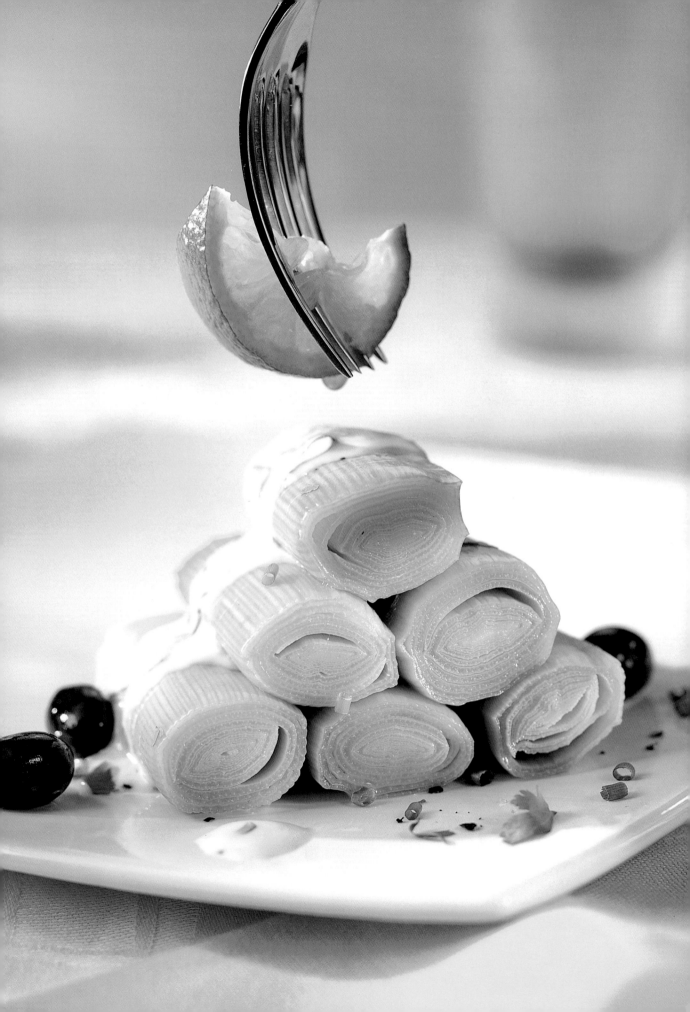

Aubergine, chickpea and coriander salad
with spicy tomato and red pepper salsa

SERVES 4

INGREDIENTS

3 large **aubergines**, cut into chunks

4 tablespoons **olive oil**

400 g/14 oz canned **chickpeas**, drained

½ teaspoon salt

2 **garlic cloves**, crushed

1 teaspoon **lemon** juice or **balsamic vinegar**

½ teaspoon **Tabasco** sauce

large bunch of **coriander**, stalks removed

warmed **pitta bread**, to serve

SPICY TOMATO AND RED PEPPER SALSA

small bunch of **coriander**, finely shredded

small bunch of **basil**, finely shredded

2–3 **garlic cloves**, chopped

1 small **red onion**, finely diced

¼ **green pepper**, neatly diced

¼ **red pepper**, neatly diced

small piece of fresh **chilli**, neatly diced

400 g/14 oz can of **tomatoes**, chopped

dash of **Tabasco** sauce

salt

Here's a perfect way to cook aubergines, not drenched in oil. Steamed lightly, they are then just brushed with oil and grilled; they come out golden brown and delicious. In striving for a lower fat cooking method these discoveries are sometimes made (someone, somewhere, will no doubt have thought of it before, but to me it was a revelation) and a well-established tradition – that aubergines need loads of oil – is overturned in a moment.

METHOD

1. Mix together all the ingredients for the salsa, season to taste, and set aside.
2. Steam the aubergines until almost tender, then toss with 3 tablespoons of the olive oil, spread on a baking sheet and brown under a preheated grill.
3. Tip the aubergines into a bowl and stir in the chickpeas, salt, garlic, lemon juice or vinegar, Tabasco, coriander and the remaining tablespoon of oil. Serve warm, with the salsa, and warmed pitta bread. Any remaining salsa can be served separately.

NUTRITIONAL INFORMATION
one serving contains

CALORIES	527
TOTAL FAT	20.3G
CARBOHYDRATES	72G
TOTAL SUGAR	12.4G
FIBRE	12.7G
SODIUM	2.6G

Timbale of pasta and roasted vegetables
with yellow and red pepper sauces

SERVES 4

INGREDIENTS

2 **red peppers**

2 **courgettes**, cut into thin ribbons

olive oil, for brushing

200 g/7 oz tiny **pasta** shapes

4 teaspoons **sun-dried tomato paste**

1 **garlic clove**, crushed

salt and pepper

YELLOW AND RED PEPPER SAUCES

1 **yellow pepper**

1 **red pepper**

2 **garlic cloves**, peeled

a few dashes of **Tabasco** sauce

salt

handful of fresh **basil** sprigs

NUTRITIONAL INFORMATION
one serving contains

CALORIES	289
TOTAL FAT	5.8G
CARBOHYDRATES	52.5G
TOTAL SUGAR	14.3G
FIBRE	5.6G
SODIUM	0.7G

A pretty way to encase a simple pasta salad. You will need to weight the timbales down: I placed small plastic tubs, filled with rice, on top of each, or you could use full jam jars. Scatter lots of small basil leaves all over the timbale and its sauces.

METHOD

1. Preheat the grill. Grill all the peppers (for the timbales and the sauce), turning frequently, until they are beginning to blacken all over. Peel and deseed the peppers and set aside. Lightly brush the courgette ribbons with oil and grill until just tender.

2. Cook the pasta in boiling water until tender. Drain well.

3. For the timbales, dice half the courgette ribbons and one red pepper. Mix with the warm pasta, the sun-dried tomato paste, garlic, salt and pepper. Cut another red pepper into 2 cm/¾ inch strips. Use alternate strips of red pepper and courgette to line four timbale dishes, ramekins or coffee cups – the strips should overlap. Press the pasta mixture into the timbales and fold over the strips of pepper and courgette. Cover the timbales with weights and leave for at least 2 hours.

4. To make the sauces, separately purée the yellow pepper and the remaining red pepper. Place each purée in a small saucepan and simmer gently with a whole garlic clove, a dash of Tabasco, a little salt and a few sprigs of basil.

5. To serve, remove the garlic and basil from the sauces. Slip the edge of a knife around the timbales to loosen them, then turn out on to four serving plates. Place a spoonful of each sauce on either side and serve at once.

Vegetable sushi

SERVES 8–10

INGREDIENTS

500 g/1 lb 2 oz **sushi** or **pudding rice**

1.2 litres/2 pints hot water

4 tablespoons **rice vinegar**

1 teaspoon **icing sugar**

3 tablespoons **tamari**

25 g/1 oz **pickled ginger**

dash of **Tabasco** sauce

1 **carrot**, cut into matchsticks

1 **courgette**, cut into matchsticks

½ **red pepper**, cut into matchsticks

1 tablespoon **olive oil**

250 g/9 oz **smoked tofu**, cut into thin strips

2 teaspoons **sesame seeds**

10 sheets of **nori seaweed**

2 tablespoons **umeboshi paste**, or
  10 **umeboshi plums**, chopped

1 small **avocado,** halved and thinly sliced

TO SERVE
tamari, pickled ginger, wasabi (optional)

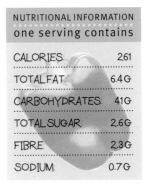

NUTRITIONAL INFORMATION one serving contains	
CALORIES	261
TOTAL FAT	6.4G
CARBOHYDRATES	41G
TOTAL SUGAR	2.6G
FIBRE	2.3G
SODIUM	0.7G

Vegetarian sushi descend easily into blandness, but with the umeboshi plums, these sushi are full of flavour. They're easier to make than they look.

METHOD

1. Put the rice in a heavy-bottomed saucepan, add the hot water, cover and bring to the boil. Reduce the heat and simmer for about 15 minutes or until all the water has evaporated and holes appear in the rice. Remove from the heat and keep in the covered pan for a further 10 minutes: the rice needs to be soft and sticky.

2. While still warm, stir in 3 tablespoons of the rice vinegar and the icing sugar. Leave to cool.

3. Mix the remaining vinegar with 2 tablespoons of tamari, the pickled ginger and the Tabasco, then divide between two small bowls. Marinate the carrot in half the mixture for 30 minutes. Add the courgette to the other bowl and marinate for 15 minutes. Add the red pepper to the carrot and marinate for 2–3 minutes.

4. Heat the oil and fry the tofu with the sesame seeds and the remaining tamari until crisp.

5. To assemble, lay a sheet of seaweed on a board. Add one-tenth of the rice and spread to the sides, leaving a 2 cm/¾ inch gap at the top and a 1 cm/½ in gap at the bottom. Keep your hands clean and wet by dipping them in warm water as you work. Using a teaspoon, spread a line of umeboshi paste (or chopped plums) along the rice, near the bottom. Add some of the vegetables and tofu, then roll upwards tightly. Moisten the seaweed at the end to seal.

6. Using a very sharp knife, trim the edges neatly, then cut each roll into eight. Serve with tamari for dipping, with pickled ginger and wasabi.

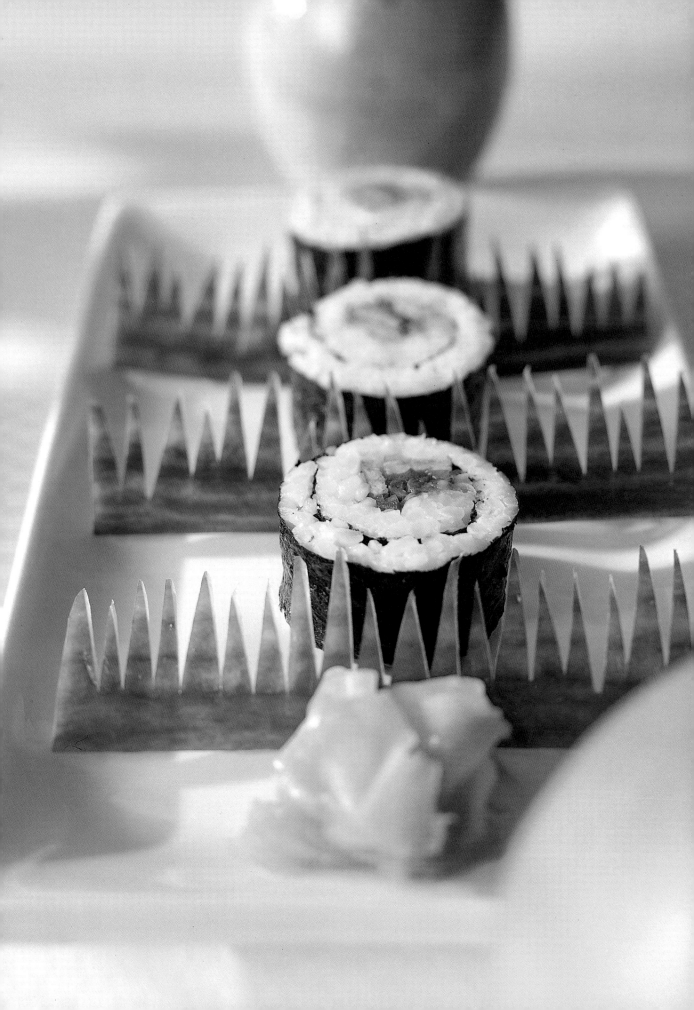

Filo purses with mushrooms and leeks
with pumpkin sauce

SERVES 4

INGREDIENTS

1 teaspoon **olive oil**

450 g/1 lb **leeks**, green parts removed, then finely sliced

1–2 **garlic cloves**, finely chopped

pinch of grated **nutmeg**

250 g/9 oz **mushrooms**, finely sliced

dash of **tamari**

dash of **Tabasco** sauce

salt and pepper

6 sheets of **filo pastry**

PUMPKIN SAUCE

500 g/1 lb 2 oz **pumpkin**, peeled and cut into chunks

½ teaspoon **mild curry paste**

½ teaspoon **bouillon powder**

¼ teaspoon **ground coriander**

¼ teaspoon salt

150 ml/5 fl oz water

Very eighties, yet very right for now: practically all the oil usually associated with filo pastry has been removed – a light spray of oil suffices. The final result is much drier but the crunchiness of the pastry has an immediate appeal. The pumpkin sauce, multiplied by four, makes a delicious soup that needs only a spoonful of yoghurt.

METHOD

1. Preheat the oven to 200°C/400°C/gas 6. Heat the oil in a large saucepan and gently sweat the leeks with the garlic and nutmeg until soft. Add the mushrooms and cook for a couple of minutes. Add the tamari, Tabasco and salt and pepper to taste, then remove from the heat.

2. Lay out the filo pastry in two piles of three sheets each, then cut in half. Place a generous heap of the vegetables in the middle of each, then lift up the pastry and twist the top to seal. Place the pastry purses on a lightly oiled baking sheet and bake for about 20 minutes, until golden and crisp.

3. Meanwhile, make the sauce. Place the pumpkin in a saucepan with the curry paste, bouillon powder, ground coriander, salt and water. Simmer for 20–25 minutes, then rub through a sieve. Taste and adjust the seasoning and serve warm, with the filo purses. Any extra sauce can be served separately or made into a soup the next day (see introduction).

NUTRITIONAL INFORMATION
one serving contains

CALORIES	219 G
TOTAL FAT	3.4 G
CARBOHYDRATES	41.7 G
TOTAL SUGAR	5.5 G
FIBRE	5.9 G
SODIUM	0.7 G

Shiitake mushroom salad
with Thai vinaigrette

SERVES 4

INGREDIENTS

1 **courgette**, diced

½ teaspoon **bouillon powder** dissolved in
 2 teaspoons water

1 teaspoon **olive oil**

200 g/7 oz **shiitake mushrooms**, sliced
 thickly

1 **garlic clove**, finely chopped

1 teaspoon **tamari**

dash of **Tabasco** sauce

1 small **Cos lettuce**, finely shredded

100 g/3½ oz **mangetout**, finely sliced

2 **spring onions**, finely sliced

THAI VINAIGRETTE

1½ tablespoons **balsamic vinegar**

4 tablespoons **rice vinegar**

1½ tablespoons **olive oil**

½ **garlic clove**, crushed

1 teaspoon **soft brown sugar**

12 **coriander seeds**, coarsely crushed

handful of fresh **coriander**, roughly chopped

1 small **red chilli**, finely chopped

As you can see, I use shiitake mushrooms often.
They are among my favourite things and so I was
happy to turn to Paul Gayler for the inspiration
behind this salad. The mushrooms are best added
warm to the salad leaves so that they absorb the
dressing ingredients.

METHOD

1. For the vinaigrette, mix the vinegars, oil, garlic,
   sugar and coriander seeds and leave to marinate
   for at least 1 hour if possible.
2. Cook the courgette with the dissolved bouillon
   powder over a high heat for 2 minutes – it
   should remain green and firm.
3. Heat the oil in a frying pan and sauté the
   mushrooms with the garlic, tamari and Tabasco
   for about 2 minutes, until just tender.
4. Pile the lettuce, mangetout and spring onions
   on to four plates. Mix the courgettes and
   mushrooms and spoon on to the lettuce. Strain
   the dressing to remove the coriander seeds, then
   stir in the fresh coriander and chilli. Spoon a
   little over the mushrooms on each plate and
   serve at once.

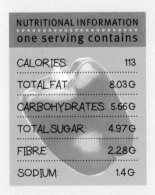

NUTRITIONAL INFORMATION one serving contains	
CALORIES:	113
TOTAL FAT:	8.03 G
CARBOHYDRATES:	5.66 G
TOTAL SUGAR:	4.97 G
FIBRE:	2.28 G
SODIUM:	1.4 G

Blinis with papaya and avocado salsa

SERVES 6

INGREDIENTS

1½ teaspoons **dried yeast**

a good pinch of sugar

150 ml/5 fl oz hand-hot water

125 g/4 oz **rye flour**

125 g/4 oz **plain flour**

½ teaspoon salt

½ beaten **egg**

150 ml/5 fl oz **milk**

2–3 tablespoons **vegetable oil** for frying

250 g/9 oz fat-free **fromage frais**, to serve

PAPAYA AND AVOCADO SALSA

1 ripe **papaya**

½ ripe **avocado**, cut into very small cubes

2 tablespoons chopped fresh **coriander**

3 cm/1 inch piece of fresh **chilli**, seeded and very
finely diced

½ teaspoon **tamarind paste**

juice of 1 **lime**

a dash of **Tabasco** sauce

freshly ground black pepper

NUTRITIONAL INFORMATION one serving contains	
CALORIES	318
TOTAL FAT	13.8 G
CARBOHYDRATES	41.3 G
TOTAL SUGAR	9.1 G
FIBRE	5.2 G
SODIUM	0.3 G

Blinis are little yeasted pancakes beloved of the Russians, who famously eat them with caviar and sour cream. I find them a perfect standby, to be topped in a hundred different ways. They are worth making in batches and freezing, then bringing back to life in a warm oven. Don't let them dry out – they need to be soft and spongy when you pop them in your mouth. Make them hardly bigger than bite size. That way you can eat loads.

The salsa has to be made shortly before serving because of the delicate avocado, which has to be very fresh.

METHOD

1. Mix the yeast with the sugar and warm water and leave in a warm place for 5–10 minutes.

2. Sift the flours together with the salt, then make a well in the centre of the flour. Add the beaten egg, milk and yeast mixture and gently mix in the flour from the edges until all the flour is combined. Cover and leave to stand in a warm place for 30–45 minutes.

3. Meanwhile, make the salsa. Slice the papaya in half and rub half through a sieve, retaining the juice. Cut the other half into very small cubes. Mix all the salsa ingredients together with the papaya juice and lime, adding Tabasco and pepper to taste.

4. Gently stir the yeast batter. Heat 1 tablespoon of oil in a heavy-based frying pan. Drop in tablespoons of the mixture and cook over a high heat for 1–2 minutes on each side. Repeat until all the blinis are cooked, adding a little more oil each time to prevent sticking. Serve warm, with the papaya salsa and some fromage frais.

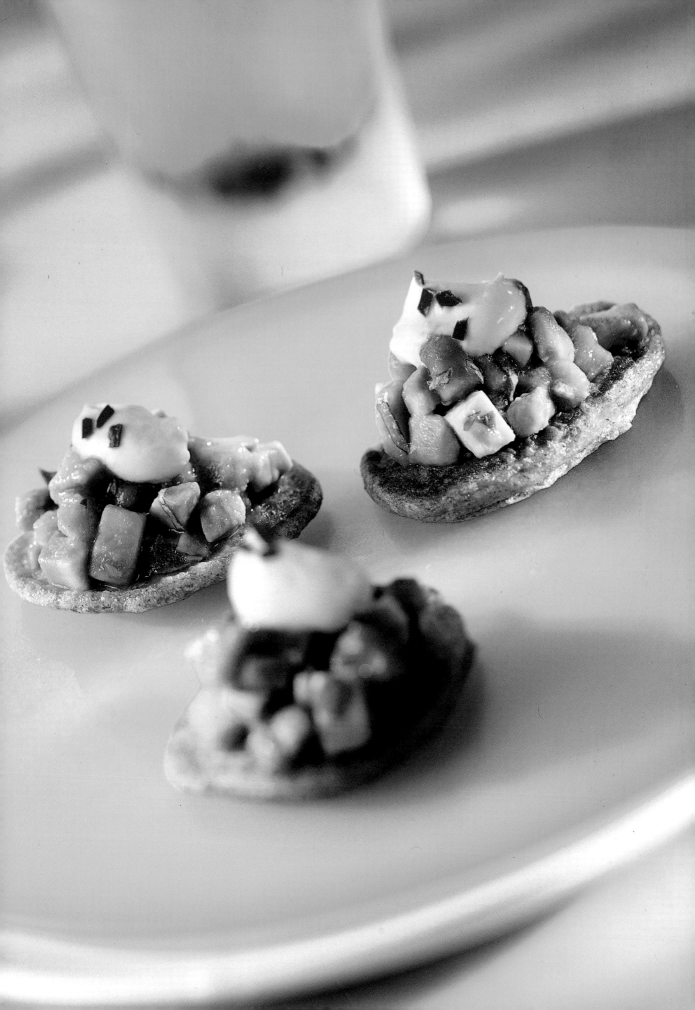

SANDWICHES, BRUSCHETTAS AND WRAPS

For working lunches and picnics, the humble **sandwich** has undergone a major revolution. Goodbye plastic bread with polystyrene cheese, hello happiness, hello artichokes and avocado, goats' cheese and watercress, wild mushrooms, peppers, enchiladas, tortillas, walnut bread and bagels. Welcome running-down-your-chin, finger-licking dressings and sauces and generous toppings. **Brilliant**.

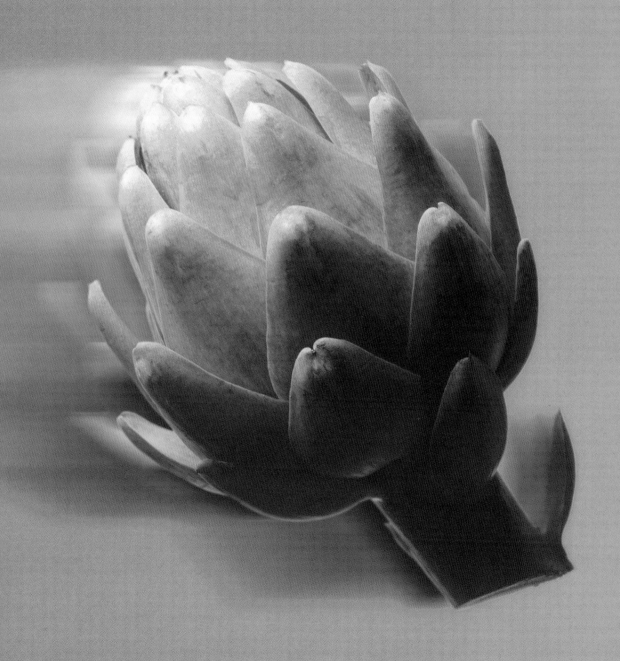

Bruschetta with roasted vegetables

SERVES 6

INGREDIENTS

1 **fennel bulb**, cut into 6 wedges

2 **courgettes**, cut diagonally into thick slices

1 **red onion**, cut into 6 pieces

1 **red pepper**, cut into 6 pieces

3 **tomatoes**, halved

1 tablespoon **olive oil**

½ teaspoon **harissa**

½ teaspoon **honey**

1 teaspoon **tamari**

1 **garlic clove**, crushed

½ teaspoon dried **marjoram**

6 slices of **sourdough bread**

sea salt

Eat this warm or cold, as a starter or light lunch with a colourful salad. The vegetables are roasted on a baking sheet with the lightest possible coating of oil – this is where spray cans of oil are really useful – then finished under the grill.

METHOD

1. Preheat the oven to 230°C/450°F/gas 8. Prepare all the vegetables. Mix the oil, harissa, honey, tamari, garlic and marjoram together, then stir in 2 tablespoons water.

2. Spray or sparingly brush a small amount of oil over a baking sheet. Put the fennel, courgettes, onion and pepper on the baking sheet and baste generously with the harissa mixture. Place in the hot oven for about 10 minutes, then add the tomatoes and roast for a further 5 minutes. Meanwhile, preheat the grill.

3. Spoon the rest of the harissa mixture over the vegetables and place the baking sheet under the hot grill for 10 minutes, or until the vegetables are tender.

4. Toast the bread on one side, turn over and rub each slice with half a roasted tomato and a little sea salt. Toast until crisp around the edges, then top with the vegetables and serve hot or cold.

NUTRITIONAL INFORMATION one serving contains	
CALORIES:	206
TOTAL FAT:	5.3 G
CARBOHYDRATES:	35.2 G
TOTAL SUGAR:	8.4 G
FIBRE:	4.6 G
SODIUM:	0.9 G

Naan bread with tikka vegetables

SERVES 6

INGREDIENTS

1 **cauliflower**, cut into small florets

250 g/9 oz **carrots**, cut into 1 cm/½ inch cubes

250 g/9 oz **courgettes**, cut into 2 cm/¾ inch cubes

2 small young **leeks**, cut into 2 cm/¾ inch thick slices

3 tablespoons **tikka paste**

200 g/7 oz low-fat **yoghurt**

6 **naan bread**

handful of fresh **coriander**

This appears in the sandwich section because it is essentially bread topped with vegetables, but in fact it is abundant enough to eat as a main meal, with lassi to drink.

METHOD

1. Preheat the oven to 200°C/400°F/gas 6. Cook the vegetables in boiling salted water for 2 minutes. Drain and refresh in cold water.

2. Coat the vegetables in the tikka paste, place on a baking sheet and roast in the hot oven for about 30 minutes, or until just cooked but still firm to the bite. Remove from the oven and mix with the yoghurt.

3. Put the naan bread in the oven for about 1 minute to warm through. Heap each naan with the vegetables, garnish with coriander and serve warm.

NUTRITIONAL INFORMATION one serving contains	
CALORIES	547
TOTAL FAT	19.8 G
CARBOHYDRATES	76.6 G
TOTAL SUGAR	17.1 G
FIBRE	7.2 G
SODIUM	1.7 G

Artichoke and avocado
with basil on marbled tomato bread

SERVES 6

INGREDIENTS

6 canned **artichoke** hearts, cut into quarters

1 tablespoon **extra-virgin olive oil**

1 large bunch of fresh **basil**, finely shredded

1 **garlic clove**, crushed

salt and freshly ground black pepper

1 **avocado**, cut into thin slices

12 slices of **marbled tomato bread**

1 tablespoon **pine nuts**, lightly toasted

200 g/7 oz mixed salad leaves, roughly chopped

This is my favourite sandwich. The artichoke hearts are better for being roasted, and of course if you can use fresh ones (as in the recipe for Asparagus and artichoke salad with wild rice on page 62) then this will be among the kings of sandwiches.

METHOD

1. Preheat the oven to 200°C/400°F/gas 6. Baste the quartered artichoke hearts with the oil and roast for about 7–8 minutes, until light brown.
2. Add the basil, garlic, salt and pepper to the roasted artichokes and sliced avocado and mix well. Divide between six of the bread slices, then scatter with the toasted pine nuts.
3. Top with a handful of mixed leaves, a little black pepper and finally the remaining slices of bread. Cut in half and eat very fresh.

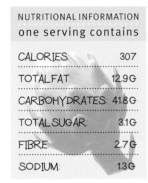

NUTRITIONAL INFORMATION
one serving contains

CALORIES:	307
TOTAL FAT:	12.9G
CARBOHYDRATES:	41.8G
TOTAL SUGAR:	3.1G
FIBRE:	2.7G
SODIUM:	1.3G

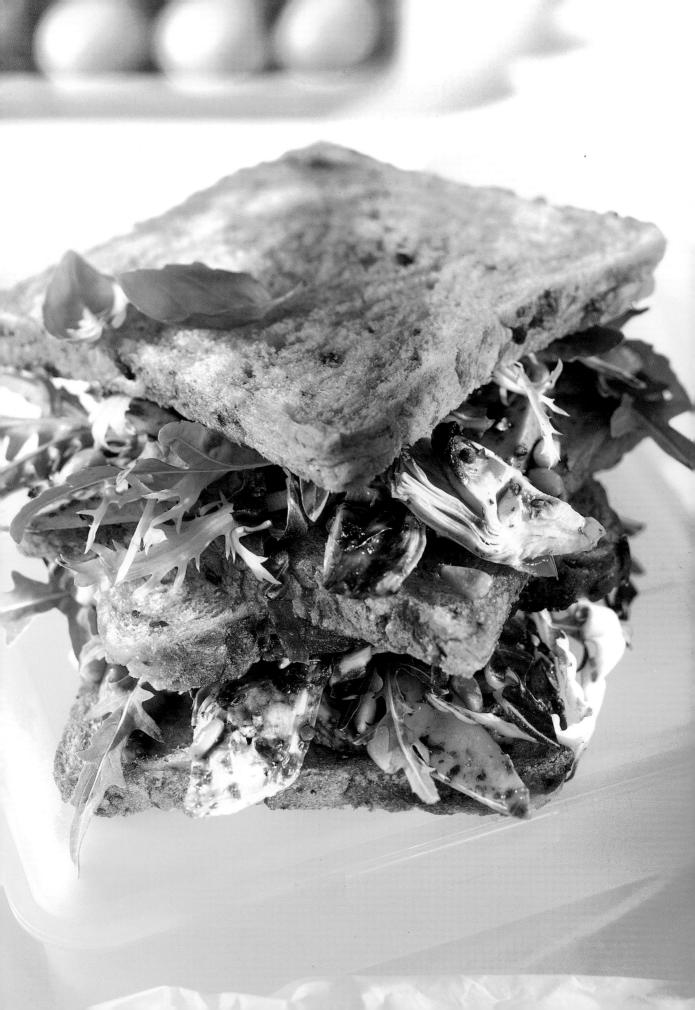

Cream cheese, sun-dried tomatoes
and spinach on rye

SERVES 6

INGREDIENTS

400 g/14 oz low-fat **soft cheese**

50 g/2 oz **sun-dried tomatoes**, soaked in
hot water, then drained and chopped

½ small **red onion**, finely chopped

¼ teaspoon ground **cumin**

salt and freshly ground black pepper

12 slices of **rye bread** (ideally half dark rye and
half light)

50 g/2 oz baby **spinach** leaves

200 g/7 oz mixed salad leaves

A real hybrid of a sandwich, which makes the most
of the culinary freedom to mix and match.

METHOD

1. Mix the soft cheese with the chopped tomatoes
   and onion and season to taste with cumin, salt
   and pepper.
2. Put the spinach on the slices of dark rye bread.
   Divide the cheese mixture between the
   sandwiches and top with the salad leaves, then
   a slice of light rye bread. Cut in half and serve.

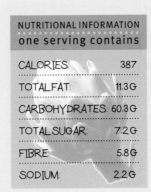

NUTRITIONAL INFORMATION one serving contains	
CALORIES:	387
TOTAL FAT:	11.3 G
CARBOHYDRATES:	60.3 G
TOTAL SUGAR:	7.2 G
FIBRE:	5.8 G
SODIUM:	2.2 G

Feta cheese sandwich
with red pepper, green beans and purple basil

SERVES 6

INGREDIENTS

125 g/4 oz **green beans**

200 g/7 oz **feta cheese**

150 g/5 oz low-fat **yoghurt**

1 **red pepper**, sliced into 5 mm/¼ inch strips

juice of ½ **lemon**

freshly ground black pepper

handful of **purple basil**, shredded

12 slices of **wholemeal** or **onion bread**

200 g/7 oz mixed salad leaves

It's good to feel the crunch in a sandwich, so keep the green beans firm and the lettuce crisp. Purple basil makes for a stunning combination of colours, but for flavour, regular green basil is fine.

METHOD

1. Cook the green beans in boiling water for about 2 minutes, then drain and refresh in cold water. Dry on kitchen paper and cut in half.
2. Crumble the feta cheese into the yoghurt. Add the red pepper strips, beans, lemon juice, black pepper and basil and mix well. Spread on to the bread and sandwich with salad leaves.

NUTRITIONAL INFORMATION one serving contains	
CALORIES:	283
TOTAL FAT:	9.3G
CARBOHYDRATES:	37.7G
TOTAL SUGAR:	6.9G
FIBRE:	5.7G
SODIUM:	2.3G

Three-mushroom wrap

SERVES 6–8

INGREDIENTS

300 g/11 oz **chestnut mushrooms**

225 g/8 oz **shiitake mushrooms**

1 tablespoon **olive oil**

25 g/1 oz **dried wild mushrooms**, soaked in
2 tablespoons hot water, 1 tablespoon tamari
and 1 tablespoon red wine

1–2 **garlic cloves**, finely chopped

1 tablespoon **tamari**

dash of **Tabasco** sauce

3–5 cm/1–2 inch piece of fresh **ginger**, grated
and squeezed

2 small **courgettes**, cut into small chunks

3 tablespoons **oyster mushroom sauce**
(or yellow bean sauce)

1 teaspoon **lemon juice**

1 teaspoon **cornflour** dissolved in 1 teaspoon
water

bunch of **basil**, shredded

small bunch of **parsley**, chopped

a sprig of **tarragon**

6–8 flat **Arabic breads**

large bunch of watercress

Here they are again, the delicious shiitake and their companion fungi. Oyster mushroom sauce is vegetarian, obviously made with the mushrooms of the same name. If you can't find it, use yellow bean sauce instead.

Be generous with the filling, arm yourself with plenty of napkins and be prepared for it to ooze out deliciously. If you can't lick your fingers after eating with them, then what is the point of being alive?

METHOD

1. Cut the chestnut and shiitake mushrooms into thick slices. Heat the oil in a large saucepan, add all the mushrooms (including the dried mushrooms' soaking liquid) and garlic and cook until softened, adding the tamari after a few minutes. Add the Tabasco and ginger juice. Add the courgettes and sauté for less than a minute, so they stay firm and green.

2. Add the oyster mushroom sauce and lemon juice and bring to the boil. Immediately add the cornflour and stir until the juices are thickened, then add the herbs.

3. Warm the breads. Spread the filling evenly over them, then lay the watercress along the centre. Fold up the bottom quarter of each bread, then roll up tightly and serve at once.

NUTRITIONAL INFORMATION one serving contains	
CALORIES:	268
TOTAL FAT:	4.1G
CARBOHYDRATES:	49.5G
TOTAL SUGAR:	2.5G
FIBRE:	2.9G
SODIUM:	2.7G

Goats' cheese and watercress
on walnut toast

SERVES 4

INGREDIENTS
1 large **tomato**, diced

4 **black olives**, finely chopped

1 teaspoon **balsamic vinegar**

freshly ground black pepper

100 g/3½ oz **goats' cheese** log, crumbled

large bunch of **watercress**, stalks removed

4 slices of **walnut bread**, lightly toasted

Assemble this moments before eating so the watercress stays crisp and sharp.

METHOD
1. Gently mix together the diced tomato, olives, vinegar and pepper. Gently fold in the goats' cheese and watercress and heap on to the bread. Serve immediately.

NUTRITIONAL INFORMATION
one serving contains

CALORIES:	178
TOTAL FAT:	6.7 G
CARBOHYDRATES:	21.9 G
TOTAL SUGAR:	2 G
FIBRE:	3.6 G
SODIUM:	1.2 G

Black bean enchilada

MAKES 10

INGREDIENTS

250 g/9 oz **black beans** (dry weight), soaked overnight

4 **garlic cloves**

2 **bay leaves**

½ **red onion**, cut into chunks

1 tablespoon **olive oil**

400 g/14 oz canned **tomatoes**

½ teaspoon **Tabasco** sauce

large bunch of fresh **coriander**, chopped

salt

1 **corn cob**, boiled until tender

1 **courgette**, diced

10 **flour tortillas**

275 ml/9 fl oz **smatana**

Use paper-thin tortillas, briefly warmed through to soften, and be generous with the salsa.

METHOD

1. Put the black beans in a saucepan with 2 whole garlic cloves, the bay leaves, onion and oil and simmer, partly covered, until the beans are half cooked (about 30 minutes).
2. Add the tomatoes, the remaining garlic (crushed), Tabasco, 2 tablespoons of the coriander and salt to taste, and simmer for a further 25–30 minutes.
3. Scrape the corn cob to remove the kernels; add the kernels to the bean mixture, along with the courgette. Simmer for a further 2 minutes.
4. Warm the tortillas briefly in the oven. Fill each one with 3 tablespoons of the bean mixture. Add 1 tablespoon of the smatana, sprinkle with fresh coriander and roll up like a pancake.

NUTRITIONAL INFORMATION
one serving contains

CALORIES:	243
TOTAL FAT:	5.3G
CARBOHYDRATES:	43.2 G
TOTAL SUGAR:	4.1G
FIBRE:	2.8G
SODIUM:	0.5G

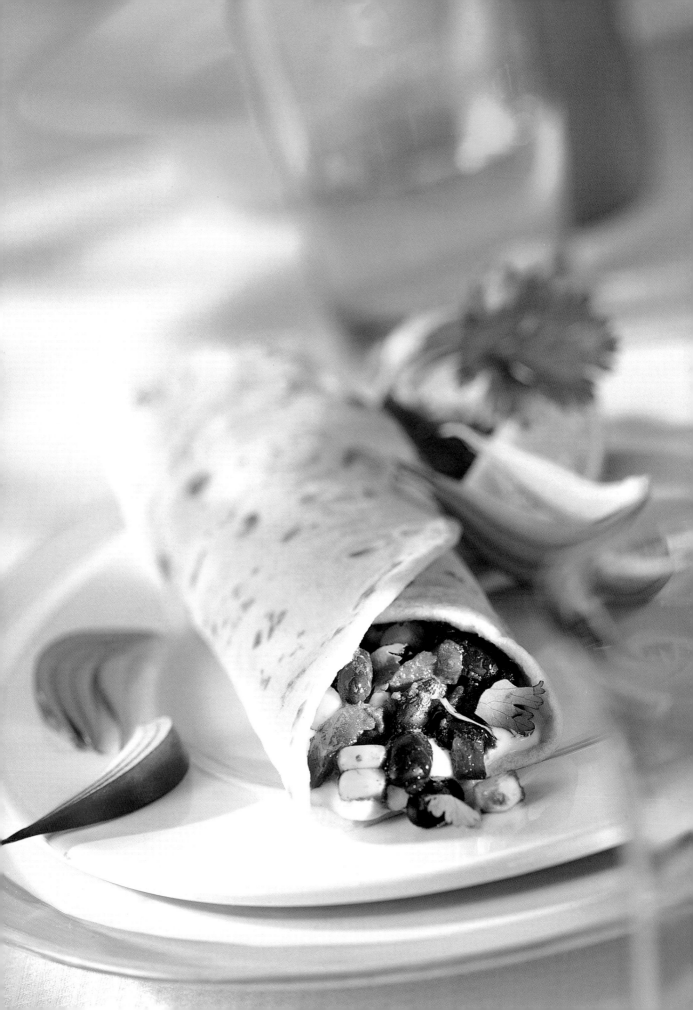

Roasted vegetables
with couscous and yoghurt in tortilla

SERVES 4

INGREDIENTS

1 **courgette**, cut on the diagonal into
  5 cm/2 inch chunks

2 **red peppers**, cut into chunks

1 **red onion**, cut into 8 wedges

2 teaspoons **olive oil**

1 **garlic clove**, crushed

dash of **Tabasco** sauce

1 teaspoon **balsamic vinegar**

salt and pepper

4 large spinach **tortillas**

200 g/7 oz young **spinach** leaves, washed
  and dried

125 g/4 oz cooked **couscous**

4 tablespoons low-fat **yoghurt**

Another fusion food sandwich, with Italian roasted vegetables in balsamic vinegar, Moroccan couscous and South American tortilla. True, there are versions of flat breads throughout the Mediterranean region, but I particularly like these paper-thin ones, especially the spinach tortillas that can be found in some supermarkets and other food shops.

METHOD

1. Preheat the oven to 200°C/400°F/gas 6. Mix the courgette, peppers and onion with the oil, garlic, Tabasco, vinegar, salt and pepper. Place in an ovenproof dish and roast in the hot oven for 35 minutes or until tender.

2. If you like, warm the tortillas for a few minutes.

3. Spread the spinach leaves over the tortillas, top with the couscous and the roasted vegetables, add a spoonful of yoghurt and roll up. Serve warm or cold.

NUTRITIONAL INFORMATION
one serving contains

CALORIES:	316
TOTAL FAT:	9.4 G
CARBOHYDRATES:	51.7 G
TOTAL SUGAR:	10.5 G
FIBRE:	4.4 G
SODIUM:	0.8 G

Blue cheese and broccoli bagels

SERVES 6

INGREDIENTS

150 g/5 oz **broccoli**, broken into small florets,
   stalks finely chopped

salt

175 g/6 oz low-fat **soft cheese**

125 g/4 oz **blue cheese** (such as Stilton),
   crumbled

40 g/1½ oz **black olives**, chopped

50 g/2 oz frozen **sweetcorn**, thawed

freshly ground black pepper

6 onion or **poppyseed bagels**

3 ripe **tomatoes**, sliced

200 g/7 oz mixed salad leaves

Now then, don't even think of eating bagels unless they are warm and fresh and smell so. However, you can cheat by sprinkling with a few drops of water and heating in a hot oven for a few minutes until they crisp up again. In fact this is something you can (and should) do with any loaf or roll.

METHOD

1. Cook the broccoli in boiling salted water for 2–3 minutes, or until just tender. Drain, refresh under cold water, then drain well.
2. Mix together the cheeses, olives and sweetcorn, and add the broccoli and pepper to taste.
3. Split the bagels and spread generously with the filling. Top with tomato slices and salad leaves.

NUTRITIONAL INFORMATION
one serving contains

CALORIES	366
TOTAL FAT	11.8G
CARBOHYDRATES	51.9G
TOTAL SUGAR	5.9G
FIBRE	3.5G
SODIUM	2.1G

Ricotta, rocket and pine nut focaccia

SERVES 4

INGREDIENTS

1 round **focaccia**

200 g/7 oz **ricotta**

200 g/7 oz **tomatoes**, sliced

about 85 g/3 oz **rocket** leaves

salt and freshly ground black pepper

15 g/½ oz **pine nuts**

25 g/1 oz **black olives**

When you have lovely, sun-ripened tomatoes and good, fresh ricotta, this sandwich emphasizes their simple, clean tastes.

METHOD

1. Slice the focaccia in half. Spread the bottom half with ricotta, then top with tomatoes, rocket, salt and pepper. Sprinkle on some pine nuts and olives.
2. Top with the other half of the focaccia, then cut into eight pieces, allowing two per person.

NUTRITIONAL INFORMATION
one serving contains

CALORIES	408
TOTAL FAT	15.5G
CARBOHYDRATES	55.3G
TOTAL SUGAR	4.7G
FIBRE	2.5G
SODIUM	2.1G

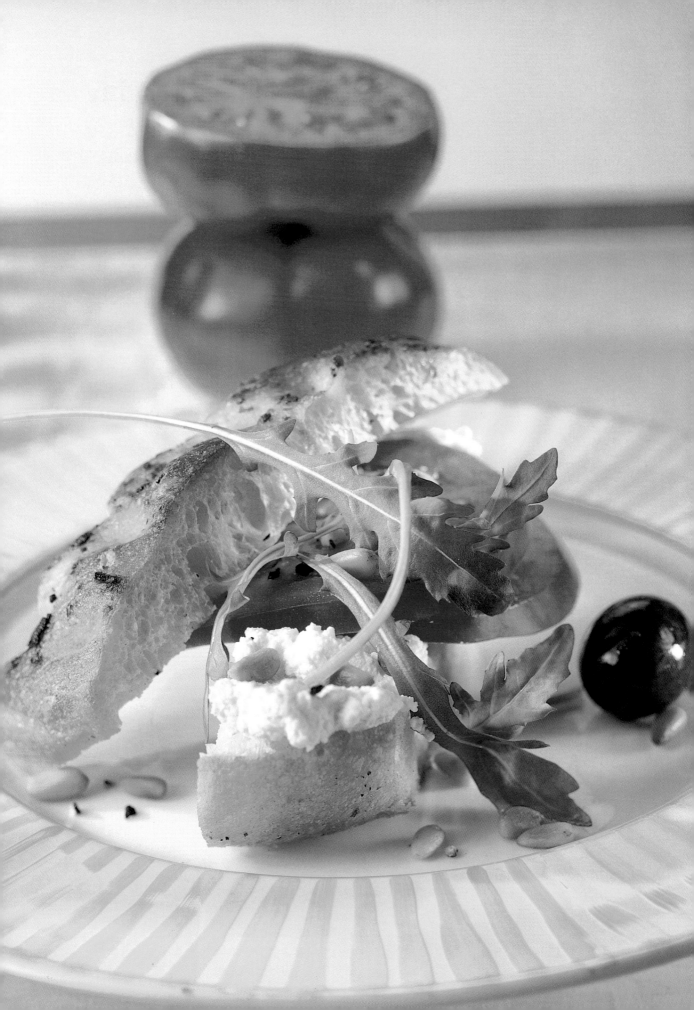

SALADS

Easily the most colourful of all foods and with the most potential for scintillating vitality and **health**. Often high in fibre and chock-full of vitamins and minerals, salads encourage chewing and the release of crucial digestive enzymes. They blast the body into action and make you full without making you fat. All this is true with one proviso. Watch out for fiendish dressings: many people's highest fat intake comes through lavish additions to their salads. Base dressings on the **low fat** versions in this book and make oil-based ones only for occasional use.

A reminder; many salad vegetables are virtually calorie-free, so even a small amount of oil in a dressing means that practically all the calories come from fat. Whether your salad is a first course or a lunch, a **good** addition to balance the meal would be a slice or two of bread, or a rice or potato salad.

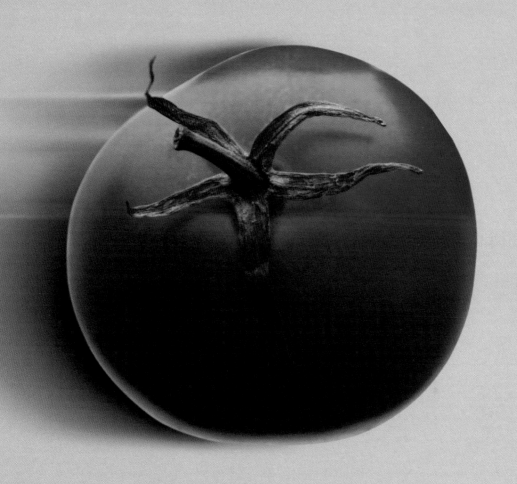

Green bean and red pepper salad
with feta cheese

SERVES 6

INGREDIENTS
2 **red peppers**

700 g/1½ lb **green beans**

200 g/7 oz **feta cheese**

French **bread**, to serve

ROASTED TOMATO DRESSING
4 **tomatoes**

2–3 whole **garlic cloves**

1 teaspoon **olive oil**

1 teaspoon **balsamic vinegar**

salt and pepper

Any salad with these three contrasting colours is bound to look stunning. Make sure the green beans are just blanched but still crisp, then immediately refreshed – essential to make the most of their forest green. Or toss immediately with the remaining ingredients and eat at once. Then the sweetness of the red pepper, the sharpness of the feta and the roasted tomato dressing make this the kind of starter you'll want to mop up with warm bread. Eat it outside in a garden, on a terrace or a patio. You are sure to be magically transported to a favourite holiday destination and you won't have had to spend the airfare.

METHOD
1. Preheat the oven to 200°C/400°F/gas 6. Preheat the grill.
2. For the dressing, put the tomatoes and garlic cloves on a small baking sheet and drizzle over the oil. Roast in the hot oven for 25–30 minutes, until the tomato skins are beginning to blacken. Put the tomatoes in a sieve over a bowl. Squeeze the garlic cloves out of their skins and add to the tomatoes. Rub the tomatoes and garlic through the sieve and stir in the balsamic vinegar. Season to taste.
3. Meanwhile, grill the red peppers until the skins begin to blacken. Leave to cool slightly, then peel and cut into strips.
4. Cook the beans in boiling salted water for 2–3 minutes. Drain and refresh under cold water, then drain well.
5. Divide the blanched beans and red pepper strips between six plates. Crumble the feta cheese over the top, then drizzle over the tomato dressing.

NUTRITIONAL INFORMATION
one serving contains

CALORIES:	298
TOTAL FAT:	10.1G
CARBOHYDRATES:	40.6G
TOTAL SUGAR:	10.1G
FIBRE:	5.1G
SODIUM:	2.2G

Three-bean and petit pois salad
with lemon and yoghurt dressing

SERVES 6

INGREDIENTS
250 g/9 oz **green beans**

250 g/9 oz frozen **broad beans**

350 g/12 oz **petit pois**

400 g/14 oz canned **butter beans**, drained

1 **spring onion**, finely chopped

LEMON AND YOGHURT DRESSING
4 **garlic cloves**, crushed

juice of ½ **lemon**

175 g/6 oz low-fat **yoghurt**

salt and pepper

½ teaspoon **wholegrain mustard**

1 tablespoon chopped fresh **chives**

Here's a new green colour scheme for that old vegetarian standby, the mixed bean salad.

METHOD
1. Blanch the green beans in boiling water for about 2 minutes. Drain, refresh in cold water, drain and set aside.
2. Cook the broad beans in boiling water for about 4 minutes and the petit pois for 2 minutes. Drain and set aside.
3. Rinse the butter beans, drain and set aside.
4. Mix together all the ingredients for the dressing, then combine with the beans. Serve sprinkled with the chopped spring onion.

NUTRITIONAL INFORMATION one serving contains	
CALORIES:	106
TOTAL FAT:	1.6 G
CARBOHYDRATES:	14.2 G
TOTAL SUGAR:	5.8 G
FIBRE:	7.6 G
SODIUM:	0.7 G

Spinach, avocado and orange salad
with orange and coriander dressing

SERVES 4

INGREDIENTS

150 g/5 oz baby **spinach**

1 small **fennel** bulb, finely sliced

2 large **oranges**, peeled and segmented

1 **avocado**, sliced

1 tablespoon **dried blueberries** (optional)

3 cm/1 inch piece of fresh mild **chilli**, very finely chopped

French **bread**, to serve

ORANGE AND CORIANDER DRESSING

1 **orange**

1 **garlic clove**, crushed

1 teaspoon **olive oil**

2 tablespoons finely chopped fresh **coriander**

a few drops of **balsamic vinegar**

2 teaspoons **teriyaki** sauce

TO SERVE

French bread

Texture, flavour, colour, vitality, this salad has it all, from the squeaky baby spinach leaves to the crunch of the fennel, the buttery avocado and the orange bursting with tangy juice.

METHOD

1. For the dressing, grate the zest from half the orange into a bowl. Squeeze the orange and add the juice to the bowl, together with all the remaining ingredients, and stir well.
2. Loosely mix the spinach, fennel, orange segments and avocado. Scatter over the blueberries and chilli. Drizzle with the dressing and serve at once.

NUTRITIONAL INFORMATION one serving contains	
CALORIES:	266
TOTAL FAT:	9.2 G
CARBOHYDRATES:	39.9 G
TOTAL SUGAR:	10.1 G
FIBRE:	5.4 G
SODIUM:	1.3 G

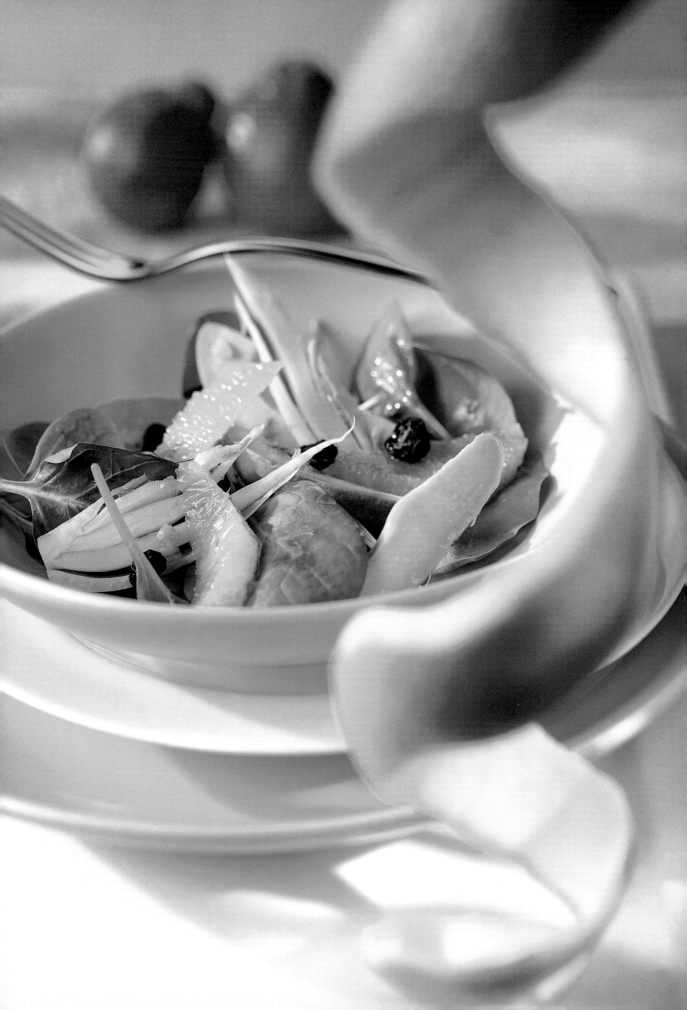

Celeriac and mixed seed salad

SERVES 6

INGREDIENTS

15 g/½ oz **sunflower seeds**

15 g/½ oz **pumpkin seeds**

1 teaspoon salt

1 small **celeriac**, shredded

150 g/5 oz **yoghurt**

1 **garlic clove**, crushed

juice of ½ **lime**

freshly ground black pepper

small handful of finely chopped fresh **parsley**
   or **coriander** (or a mixture of both)

French **bread**, to serve

Because I really was convinced that celeriac needed copious quantities of mayonnaise, I had almost relegated it to the shelf, at least as far as salads are concerned. But as it is one of my favourite vegetables, I persevered and came up with this salad, which is full of celeriac's other great friend – lemon juice. The dry toasted seeds do it great justice.

METHOD

1. Heat a heavy-based frying pan, add the seeds and salt and roast over a low heat, stirring frequently, until they start to pop. Remove from the heat and set aside.

2. Toss the celeriac with the remaining ingredients, including most of the seeds, but reserving some to sprinkle over the salad just before serving. Serve with bread, and some mixed salad leaves.

NUTRITIONAL INFORMATION one serving contains	
CALORIES:	208
TOTAL FAT:	4.8 G
CARBOHYDRATES:	34.5 G
TOTAL SUGAR:	4.3 G
FIBRE:	3.7 G
SODIUM:	1.2 G

Kohlrabi and yellow pepper salad
with a grain mustard dressing

SERVES 4

INGREDIENTS

2 heads of **kohlrabi,** peeled and thinly sliced

1 large yellow or **orange pepper**, cut into
    4 cm/1½ inch squares

2 small heads of **chicory**, quartered

GRAIN MUSTARD DRESSING

1 **garlic clove**, crushed

1 tablespoon **olive oil**

2 teaspoons **wholegrain mustard**

1 teaspoon **balsamic vinegar**

dash of **tamari**

If you've ever wondered what to do with kohlrabi, try this salad. It's beautifully simple to make and is a brilliant source of folic acid and vitamin C.

METHOD

1. Blanch the kohlrabi in boiling water for less than 1 minute. Drain, refresh in cold water, then drain and leave to cool.

2. Mix together all the ingredients for the dressing, then toss with the salad vegetables and leave for 10 minutes before serving.

NUTRITIONAL INFORMATION
one serving contains

CALORIES:	148
TOTAL FAT:	5.1G
CARBOHYDRATES:	19.2G
TOTAL SUGAR:	17.7G
FIBRE:	10G
SODIUM:	0.2

Asparagus and artichoke salad
with wild rice and basil dressing

SERVES 4

INGREDIENTS

125 g/4 oz **wild rice**

4 globe **artichokes**

juice of 1 **lemon**

1 large bunch of **asparagus**

1 tablespoon **olive oil**

1 tablespoon **lime juice**

1 **garlic clove**, crushed

salt and pepper

¼ **red pepper**, finely diced

BASIL DRESSING

1 tablespoon **wholegrain mustard**

handful of fresh **basil**, shredded

1 tablespoon **olive oil**

1 **garlic clove**, crushed

juice of ½ **lemon**

salt and pepper

To me, wild rice has to have exploded, its tough outer husk torn apart by the cooking process. So-called al dente, it is harsh on the stomach and impossible on the teeth. So cook it a very long time – at least 45 minutes – and discover why it is called the caviar of grains.

METHOD

1. Cook the wild rice for about 45 minutes, or until soft and the grains are bursting. Drain well.

2. While the rice is cooking, trim the artichokes and add to a large saucepan of boiling water with the lemon juice. Boil for 25 minutes, or until tender. Refresh in cold water and leave to drain upside down. Remove the outer leaves and any woody stalk and scrape out the hairy 'choke'. Cut into wedges.

3. Blanch the asparagus in boiling water for 1–2 minutes or until just tender, depending on its thickness. Refresh in cold water and drain well.

4. Mix together all the ingredients for the basil dressing and set aside.

5. Preheat the grill. Mix together the olive oil, lime juice, garlic, 1 tablespoon water, salt and pepper and toss the artichokes and asparagus in this mixture. Grill until lightly charred. Toss the grilled vegetables with the rice and the basil dressing. Garnish with diced red pepper.

NUTRITIONAL INFORMATION one serving contains	
CALORIES:	243
TOTAL FAT:	9.3G
CARBOHYDRATES:	32.1G
TOTAL SUGAR:	4.9G
FIBRE:	1.6G
SODIUM:	0.8G

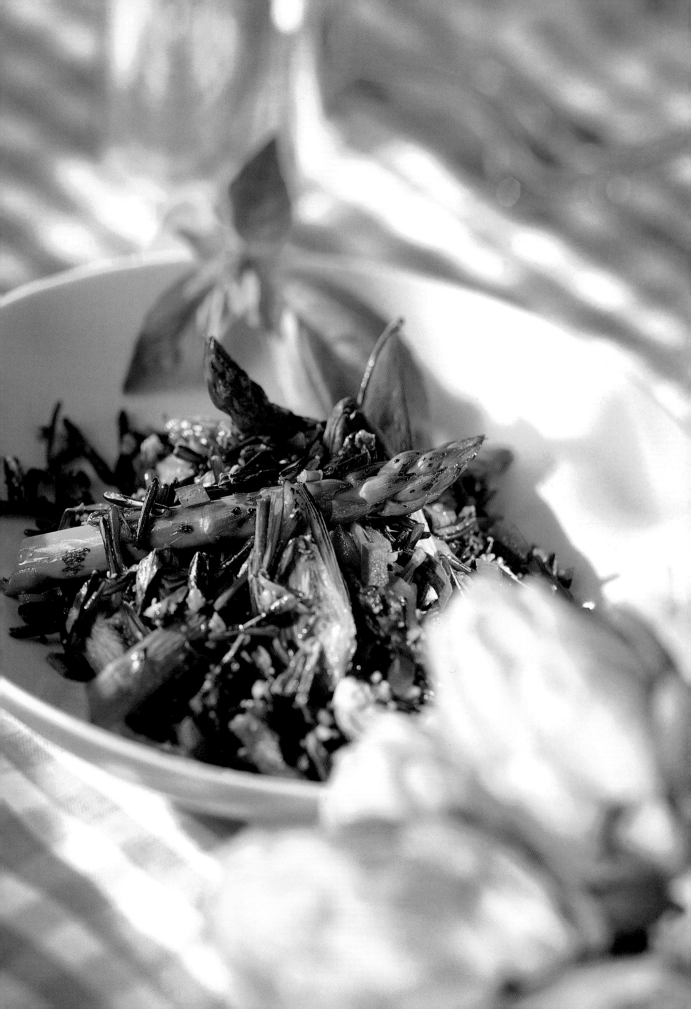

Five-grain salad
with carrots and courgettes

SERVES 8

INGREDIENTS

200 g/7 oz **wheat grains**, soaked overnight

200 g/7 oz **spelt**

200 g/7 oz **brown rice**

200 g/7 oz **barley**

3 tablespoons **olive oil**

200 g/7 oz **buckwheat**

1 **red onion**, chopped

juice of 2 **lemons**

1 **garlic clove**, crushed

½ teaspoon salt and ½ teaspoon freshly ground
black pepper

25 g/1 oz fresh **parsley**, finely chopped

1 large **carrot**, cut into julienne strips

1 large **courgette**, cut into julienne strips

1 **avocado**, sliced

Whole wheat grains, sometimes called wheat berries, are sold in health food shops, as are buckwheat and spelt (which is a species of wheat). If you can't get hold of one or other of the grains, simply increase the quantities of other grains.
For the perfect contrast of colour and flavour, serve this with a simple tomato and black olive salad.

METHOD

1. Cook the wheat, spelt, brown rice and barley in plenty of boiling water for about 45 minutes, or until tender. Drain well.

2. Heat 1 tablespoon of the oil in a saucepan, add the buckwheat and sauté until it pops. Add just enough boiling water to cover the grains, bring to the boil and simmer for about 15 minutes, until the liquid has been absorbed and the grains are tender.

3. Heat the remaining oil and sauté the onion until tender. Remove from the heat and stir in the lemon juice, 2 tablespoons water, garlic, salt, pepper and parsley.

4. Put all the grains in a large bowl and pour the dressing over. Mix well, then stir in the carrot, courgette and avocado.

NUTRITIONAL INFORMATION
one serving contains

CALORIES:	557
TOTAL FAT:	12.9G
CARBOHYDRATES:	105G
TOTAL SUGAR:	3.1G
FIBRE:	3.2G
SODIUM:	0.3G

Potato and green bean salad
with a roasted tomato dressing

SERVES 2

INGREDIENTS
250 g/9 oz waxy **potatoes**, cut into small
chunks

1 **red onion**, cut into thin rings

100 g/3½ oz **green beans**

ROASTED TOMATO AND OLIVE DRESSING
4 ripe **tomatoes**

1 teaspoon **olive oil** (or oil from a jar of sun-
dried tomatoes)

1 **garlic clove**, crushed

sea salt and freshly ground black pepper

5 large **black olives**, finely chopped

Choose waxy potatoes such as Pink Fir Apple,
Charlotte or Jersey Royal and dress while they are
still warm. As an alternative to the onion, you
could include a couple of sticks of celery, sliced
quite thinly.

METHOD
1. Preheat the oven to 200°C/400°F/gas 6.
2. For the dressing, put the tomatoes on a small
   baking sheet and drizzle over the oil. Roast in
   the hot oven for 25–30 minutes, until they are
   beginning to shrivel and blacken in places.
   Leave to cool slightly. Blend, then rub the
   tomatoes through a sieve into a bowl. Add the
   garlic, and salt and pepper to taste. Stir in the
   chopped olives.
3. While the tomatoes are roasting, boil the
   potatoes in salted water for about 10 minutes
   or until tender. Drain well and place in a serving
   bowl. Add the onion rings. Spoon the tomato
   dressing over the potatoes and leave for about
   20 minutes for the flavours to marry.
4. Cook the beans in boiling salted water for 2–3
   minutes. Drain and refresh under cold water,
   then drain well. To serve, add the beans to the
   salad bowl and toss gently.

NUTRITIONAL INFORMATION
one serving contains

CALORIES:	188
TOTAL FAT:	4.7 G
CARBOHYDRATES:	32.7 G
TOTAL SUGAR:	10 G
FIBRE:	5.5 G
SODIUM:	1.1 G

Super healthy layered salad

SERVES 4

INGREDIENTS

85 g/3 oz **wild rice**

150 g/5 oz **brown rice**

3 tablespoons **olive oil**

3 tablespoons fresh **lime juice**

1½ tablespoons **tamari**

2 teaspoons **seaweed** (nori) flakes

4 tablespoons mixed **bean sprouts**, including lentil, mung bean

4 tablespoons cooked **chickpeas**

2 tablespoons toasted **sunflower seeds**

2 tablespoons toasted **sesame seeds**

1 **red pepper**, cut into small dice

150 g/5 oz **mangetout**, blanched in boiling water for 1 minute, refreshed, and sliced on the diagonal

Each of the ingredients contributes its own package of vitamins and minerals in this wonderfully nutritious lunch.

METHOD

1. Cook the wild rice and the brown rice separately in boiling water until tender.
2. Drain, then mix both types of rice together with the olive oil, lime juice, tamari and nori flakes, and place in a serving dish.
3. Sprinkle with the bean sprouts, then the chickpeas, then the seeds, then the diced red pepper, and finally the mangetout. Serve at once.

NUTRITIONAL INFORMATION
one serving contains

CALORIES	706
TOTAL FAT	23.9 G
CARBOHYDRATES	107 G
TOTAL SUGAR	8 G
FIBRE	6.8 G
SODIUM	2 G

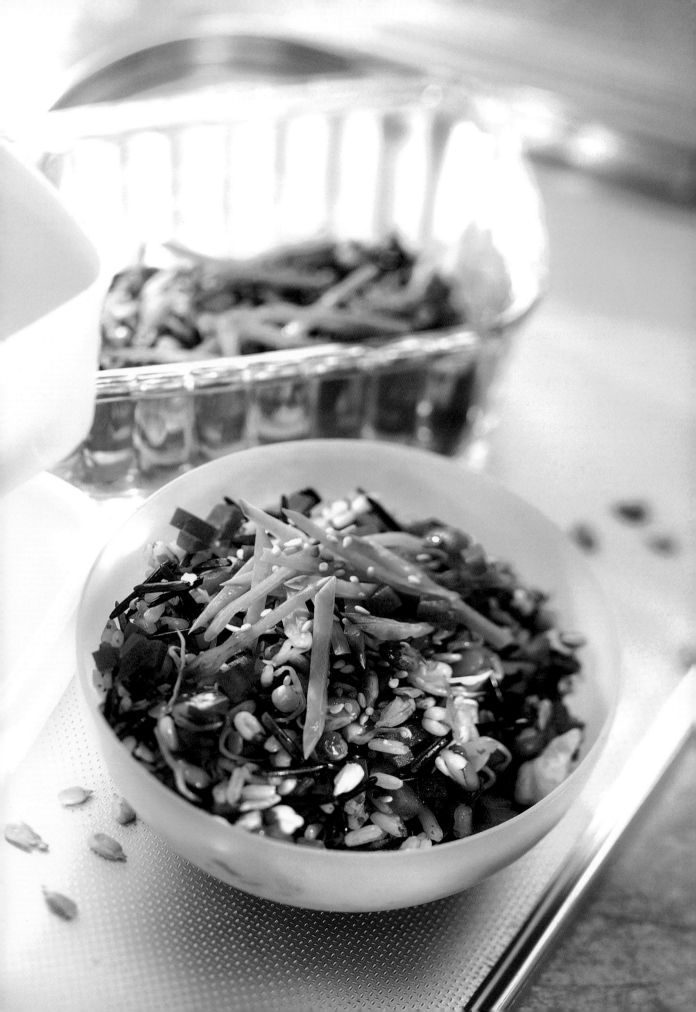

Warm pasta salad
with sun-dried tomato dressing

SERVES 4

INGREDIENTS

200 g/7 oz **mushrooms**, sliced

½ teaspoon **olive oil**

1 **red pepper**

500 g/1 lb 2 oz **penne** pasta

1 tablespoon freshly grated **Parmesan** cheese
(optional)

SUN-DRIED TOMATO DRESSING

85 g/3 oz **sun-dried tomatoes** (ready-to-eat
but not preserved in oil)

175 g/6 oz **yoghurt**

freshly ground black pepper

½ teaspoon **caster sugar**

2 tablespoons chopped fresh **basil**

Serve this warm, to bring out the sunny flavours of the pepper, tomatoes and basil.

METHOD

1. For the dressing, put all the ingredients into a blender with 150 ml/5 fl oz water and blend until smooth. Set aside.
2. Preheat the grill. Put the mushrooms in a bowl, drizzle over the olive oil and toss to coat the mushrooms. Put the pepper and mushrooms under the grill, turning the pepper frequently. Remove the mushrooms when they are tender. Remove the pepper when it is blackened on all sides. Leave to cool slightly, then peel and cut into 12 thick slices.
3. Meanwhile, cook the pasta until it is just tender, then drain.
4. Toss the pasta with the pepper and mushrooms and the dressing and serve at once, sprinkled with Parmesan if you like.

NUTRITIONAL INFORMATION
one serving contains

CALORIES:	403
TOTAL FAT:	15.8G
CARBOHYDRATES:	55G
TOTAL SUGAR:	8.6G
FIBRE:	3.6G
SODIUM:	0.8G

Sweet potato, avocado, tofu
and mixed leaf salad with baby plum tomatoes

SERVES 4

INGREDIENTS

125 g/4 oz **tofu**, cut into thick strips

3 tablespoons **teriyaki** sauce

2 tablespoons **yellow bean** sauce

2 tablespoons **olive oil**

1 tablespoon **wholegrain mustard**

1 teaspoon **balsamic vinegar**

2 **sweet potatoes**, baked, peeled and sliced

1 ripe **Hass avocado**, peeled and thinly sliced

125 g/4 oz **baby plum** or **cherry tomatoes**

250 g/9 oz mixed salad leaves, including some
   coriander and rocket

Here's a really intriguing mix of flavours, which I have served as a first course to great acclaim.

METHOD

1. Preheat the oven to 200°C/400°F/gas 6. Marinate the tofu in the teriyaki and yellow bean sauce for about 20 minutes, then roast for 15 minutes.

2. Mix the olive oil, mustard and vinegar together, then gently toss with the sweet potatoes, avocado, tomatoes and tofu. Serve on a bed of mixed leaves.

NUTRITIONAL INFORMATION
one serving contains

CALORIES:	431
TOTAL FAT:	17.5G
CARBOHYDRATES:	63.6G
TOTAL SUGAR:	18.8G
FIBRE:	9.1G
SODIUM:	2.6G

Egg thread noodle salad

SERVES 4–6

INGREDIENTS

200 g/7 oz fresh **spinach** leaves

⅓ of a **cucumber**, peeled

1 teaspoon **rice vinegar**

250 g/9 oz thread **egg noodles**

1 tablespoon **olive oil**

100 g/3½ oz **mangetout**

4 **spring onions**, sliced diagonally

1 teaspoon **tamari**

dash of **Tabasco** sauce

3 small heads of **Little Gem lettuce**

1 **red pepper**, finely sliced

1 tablespoon toasted **sesame seeds**

small bunch of **coriander**, separated into sprigs

1 cm/½ inch piece of fresh **chilli**, diced

TERIYAKI DRESSING

125 ml/4 fl oz **teriyaki** sauce

125 g/4 oz **yellow bean** sauce

juice of 1 **lime**

1 stalk of **lemongrass**, very finely chopped

5 cm/2 inch piece of fresh **ginger**, grated

NUTRITIONAL INFORMATION
one serving contains

CALORIES	404
TOTAL FAT	11.8 G
CARBOHYDRATES	60.5 G
TOTAL SUGAR	12.6 G
FIBRE	6.2 G
SODIUM	7.5 G

Go to any Japanese, Thai or Chinese supermarket and you will find almost as many different types of noodles as you would pastas in an Italian deli. There are egg and rice noodles of several thicknesses, soba (buckwheat) noodles, udon noodles – thick, pale and slippery – and wiry, transparent 'cellophane' soya noodles. You begin to understand why it is thought that pasta originated in the east and not in Italy. Most, apart from soba, take considerably less time to cook than conventional pastas. Refresh the noodles thoroughly in cold water so that they are not in the least bit sticky and loosen them with two forks before mixing with the other ingredients.

METHOD

1. Wash the spinach and place in a saucepan over medium heat until it just wilts. Leave to chill.
2. Cut the cucumber into thin batons and toss with the rice vinegar. Set aside.
3. Cook the noodles according to the packet instructions. Refresh thoroughly in cold water, drain and set aside.
4. Heat the oil in a large nonstick pan. Add the mangetout and spring onions, tamari and Tabasco and stir-fry over a high heat for about 20 seconds.
5. Mix all the ingredients for the dressing, squeezing in the juice from the ginger. Combine the dressing with the noodles and the stir-fried mangetout mixture.
6. To serve, separate the lettuce leaves and divide between the serving plates. Twist the noodles with a large fork and place on the lettuce. Scatter over the wilted spinach, cucumber batons, red pepper strips, sesame seeds, coriander and chilli and serve at once.

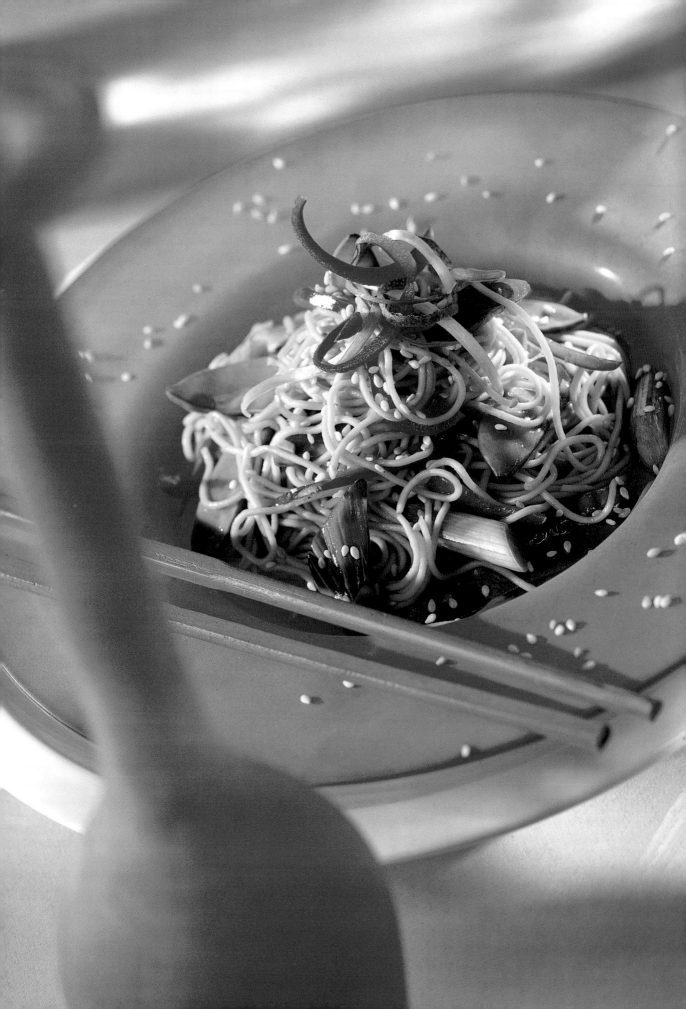

Ricotta quenelles
with watercress and cherry tomatoes

SERVES 6

INGREDIENTS

250 g/9 oz **ricotta**

1 **garlic clove**, crushed

sea salt and freshly ground black pepper

5–6 large **basil leaves**, shredded

2 large bunches of **watercress**

300 g/11 oz **cherry tomatoes**, cut in half

French **bread**, to serve

ROASTED TOMATO AND OLIVE DRESSING

4 ripe **tomatoes**

1 teaspoon **olive oil** (or oil from a jar of
    sun-dried tomatoes)

1 **garlic clove**, crushed

sea salt and freshly ground black pepper

5 large **black olives**, finely chopped

Choose your watercress carefully, preferably not in plastic sachets where it weeps pathetically and comes out limp, flaccid and yellowed around the gills. Some places do still sell big, juicy bunches with peppery leaves and this is what you need for this salad. You'll find that it sits proudly on the plate and doesn't immediately collapse into a disappointing nothingness. Watercress contains lots of iron, which is good for the blood.

METHOD

1. Preheat the oven to 200°C/400°F/gas 6. For the dressing, put the tomatoes on a small baking sheet and drizzle over the oil. Roast in the hot oven for 25–30 minutes, until they are beginning to shrivel and blacken in places. Leave to cool slightly. Blend briefly, then rub through a sieve into a bowl. Add the garlic, and salt and pepper to taste. Stir in the olives.

2. Mix the ricotta with the garlic, salt, pepper and basil. Shape the ricotta mixture into quenelles, using two teaspoons.

3. Arrange the watercress and cherry tomatoes on six plates, together with 3–4 ricotta quenelles. Drizzle the dressing over the salad.

NUTRITIONAL INFORMATION
one serving contains

CALORIES:	243G
TOTAL FAT:	7.8G
CARBOHYDRATES:	34.6G
TOTAL SUGAR:	5.3G
FIBRE:	2.4G
SODIUM:	1.5G

Spinach, mango and smoked tofu salad

SERVES 6

INGREDIENTS
275 g/10 oz **smoked tofu**, cut into thin strips

1 tablespoon **olive oil**

1 tablespoon **tamari**

1 tablespoon **sesame seeds**

300 g/11 oz fresh baby **spinach** leaves

225 g/8 oz moist dried **mango**, cut into thin slivers

French **bread**, to serve

MANGO DRESSING
150 ml/5 fl oz **mango juice**

1 tablespoon **olive oil**

1 tablespoon **tamari**

½ teaspoon **balsamic vinegar**

dash of **Tabasco** sauce

freshly ground black pepper

If you cannot find the moist, ready-to-eat dried mangoes with no hint of crystallized sugar, then use a fresh mango instead. Cut it into slices and sear it in a dry nonstick pan until it browns around the edges. Leave it to cool or serve it just warm and added to the salad at the last moment.

METHOD
1. Sauté the smoked tofu with the olive oil, tamari and sesame seeds until crisp and browned, adding 1 tablespoon water to prevent sticking.
2. To make the dressing, put all the ingredients into a bowl and whisk together.
3. Divide the spinach leaves between six plates and scatter the mango and smoked tofu on top. Serve the dressing separately.

NUTRITIONAL INFORMATION one serving contains	
CALORIES:	328
TOTAL FAT:	9.8 G
CARBOHYDRATES:	50.2 G
TOTAL SUGAR:	20.6 G
FIBRE:	4.8 G
SODIUM:	1.8 G

Cheat's pickled vegetables

SERVES 6–8

INGREDIENTS

½ **mooli**, cut into 2 cm/¾ inch squares

3 **carrots**, cut on a slant

1 **cauliflower**. separated into small florets

100 g/3½ oz **green beans**, topped and tailed

1 **cucumber**, cut in half lengthways, seeds
   removed and cut into 5 mm/¼ inch half-moons

175 ml/6 fl oz **rice vinegar**, white wine vinegar
   or cider vinegar

1 teaspoon **caster sugar**

3 cm/1 inch piece of fresh **ginger**, grated and
   squeezed

8 **juniper berries**, slightly crushed

TO SERVE (OPTIONAL)

2 teaspoons toasted **sesame seeds**

1–2 teaspoons **seaweed** (nori) flakes

85 g/3 oz cracked **black** and **green olives**

Pickled vegetables usually need to be bottled in airtight jars and are not ready for consumption for a few days. I can never think that far ahead, so this is a quick version. The vegetables can still be kept for several days. An umeboshi plum (pickled Japanese plums, available from all Japanese stores and most wholefood shops) in the pickling medium adds a perfect sour note. The nutritional analysis includes the sesame seeds. Nori seaweed contains very little fat, but olives would nudge up the fat content slightly.

METHOD

1. Briefly blanch the mooli, carrots, cauliflower and green beans in separate saucepans of boiling water – they should take less than 1 minute each. Drain and refresh briefly in cold water (they should still be warm when the vinegar is added). Place all the vegetables in a large bowl, together with the cucumber.

2. Mix the vinegar, sugar, ginger juice and juniper berries and pour over the vegetables. Cover and leave in the refrigerator for at least 2 hours and up to 3–4 days.

3. To serve, scatter over the olives, or sprinkle with sesame seeds and nori flakes.

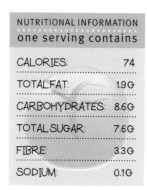

NUTRITIONAL INFORMATION one serving contains	
CALORIES:	74
TOTAL FAT:	1.9G
CARBOHYDRATES:	8.6G
TOTAL SUGAR:	7.6G
FIBRE:	3.3G
SODIUM:	0.1G

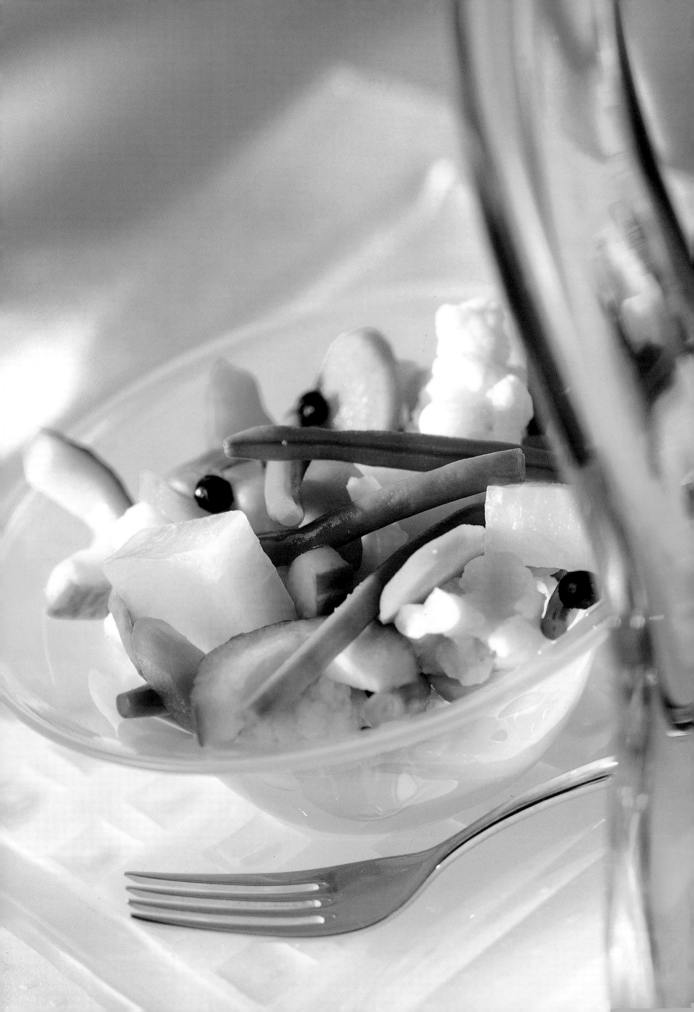

MAIN COURSES

Time was when three **square meals** a day was the norm, with three courses to at least two of them. For most people now, one meal a day at most contains what might be described as a main course and this is mostly eaten in the evenings. A main course is where you let go, replenish and **nourish** yourself physically, emotionally. To meet not only common sense but also nutritional guidelines, make the dish predominantly **carbohydrate** – or serve with rice, noodles, potatoes or bread as suggested in many of the recipes – and **go easy** on the fat.

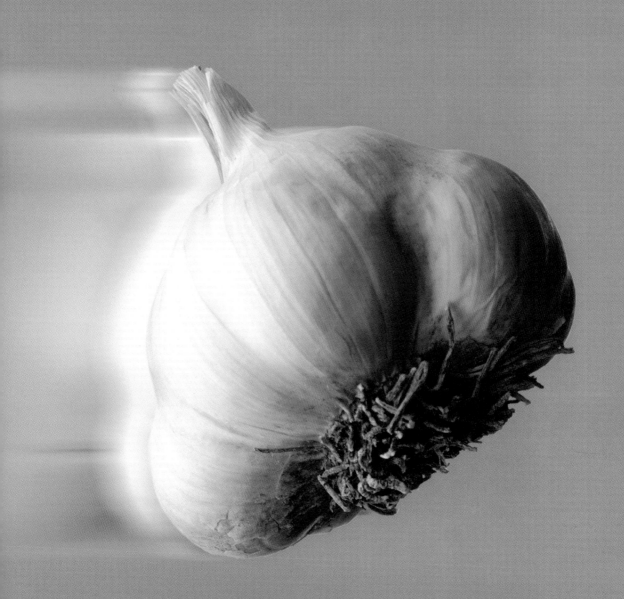

Spiced Puy lentils
with roasted vegetables

SERVES 6

INGREDIENTS

500 g/1 lb 2 oz **Puy lentils**

1 **red onion**, cut into chunks

3–6 **garlic cloves**, finely sliced

1 unwaxed **lemon**, cut into 8 pieces

1 **bay leaf**

2 tablespoons ground **cumin**

1 teaspoon ground **coriander**

6–7 **saffron** threads

5 cm/2 inch piece of **red chilli**, finely chopped

1 teaspoon **mustard**

handful each of fresh **basil**, **coriander** and **parsley**, roughly chopped

200 g/7 oz fresh **spinach**, roughly chopped

1 teaspoon **tamari**

brown **rice** or mashed potatoes, to serve

ROASTED VEGETABLES

3 small **courgettes**, cut into large chunks

3 large **carrots**, cut into large chunks

1 large **red onion**, cut into large chunks

3 tablespoons **olive oil**

salt and freshly ground black pepper

Puy lentils hold their shape even when tender; you should cook them until the lemon is meltingly soft, when it is delicious and reminiscent of Moroccan dishes. You can serve the stew on its own or with mashed potatoes or brown rice for a wintry main course. The lentils are a great source of protein and are virtually fat free.

METHOD

1. Heat the oven to its highest setting.

2. Put the lentils in a saucepan, together with the onion, garlic, lemon, bay leaf, cumin, coriander, saffron, chilli and mustard. Cover with cold water, bring to the boil, then reduce the heat and simmer for about 20 minutes. Add a further 900 ml/1½ pints water and simmer for about 10 more minutes, until tender.

3. Meanwhile, for the roasted vegetables, mix the courgettes, carrots and onion with the oil, salt and pepper, spread on a baking sheet and bake for 35–40 minutes, until tender.

4. Add the roasted vegetables to the lentils with half the chopped herbs; simmer for 15 minutes.

5. To serve, add the remaining herbs, the spinach and tamari and season to taste with salt and pepper. Serve at once, with rice or potatoes.

NUTRITIONAL INFORMATION one serving contains	
CALORIES:	405
TOTAL FAT:	11.6 G
CARBOHYDRATES:	66.5 G
TOTAL SUGAR:	10.5 G
FIBRE:	8 G
SODIUM:	0.6 G

Roasted Jerusalem artichokes
with fennel and red onion

SERVES 4

INGREDIENTS

500 g/1 lb 2 oz **Jerusalem artichokes,**
   scrubbed and sliced

2 small **fennel bulbs**, cut into quarters
   (or 1 large bulb, cut into 8 pieces)

2 whole heads of **garlic**, sliced in half

1 large **red onion**, cut into 6

2 teaspoons **tamarind paste**

1 tablespoon **tamari**

juice of ½ **lime**

3 tablespoons **olive oil**

1 tablespoon hot water

salt and pepper

4 fresh mild **chillies**

new **potatoes**, boiled in their skins, to serve

If sweet, mild chillies are not available, use a red pepper, cut into quarters and added 10 minutes before the end of cooking time. The chillies look pretty, but don't eat them unless you can take the heat. Should the juices dry out when roasting, baste with a little more hot water or stock, turning the vegetables often so they don't burn. Eat when very tender.

METHOD

1. Preheat the oven to 180°C/350°F/gas 4.
2. Par-boil the artichokes for 3 minutes. Drain and add to the fennel, garlic and onion. Mix the remaining ingredients (except the chillies) and gently toss with the vegetables to coat them in the mixture. Place in a roasting tin and roast for 15 minutes, then increase the oven temperature to 200°C/400°F/gas 6 and roast for a further 25 minutes, adding the chillies for the last 10 minutes only.
3. Serve hot, with half a head of roasted garlic per person, and a helping of new potatoes.

NUTRITIONAL INFORMATION
one serving contains

CALORIES	380
TOTAL FAT	12.6G
CARBOHYDRATES	62.5G
TOTAL SUGAR	11.9G
FIBRE	12.6G
SODIUM	1G

Stir-fried broccoli, mushrooms,
cashew nuts and water chestnuts with egg noodles

SERVES 6

INGREDIENTS

500 g/1 lb 2 oz cooked **egg noodles**

1½ tablespoons **sunflower oil**

1 large head of **broccoli**, cut into 2 cm/¾ inch
   florets

500 g/1 lb 2 oz each of **button** and **shiitake
   mushrooms**

4 tablespoons **water chestnuts**

1 tablespoon **tamari**

4 tablespoons **teriyaki** sauce

1 small fresh **chilli**, finely chopped

1–2 tablespoons **cashew nuts**, toasted in a dry
   pan with a little salt

salt and pepper

Adding one or two special ingredients such as cashew nuts and water chestnuts turns a simple stir-fry into a rather grand one. Spring onions, cut on the diagonal and seared in the pan, make an appropriate garnish. This stir-fry can also be served cold, as a salad, in which case you should rinse the cooked noodles in plenty of cold water so they don't become sticky. A light but filling lunch, this comes in at a fraction over the 'magic' 40% of its calories from fat – but it still has only 7 g of fat per serving.

METHOD

1. Cook the noodles in boiling water, drain and set aside.

2. Heat the oil in a large wok until hot. Throw in the broccoli florets and sauté for 1 minute, adding a drop of water if necessary. Add the mushrooms and sauté for a further 2–3 minutes. Finally add the water chestnuts, tamari and teriyaki sauce, stir briskly, then remove from the heat.

3. Stir in the chilli and cashew nuts, season to taste and mix with the cooked noodles. Eat hot or cold.

NUTRITIONAL INFORMATION
one serving contains

CALORIES:	159
TOTAL FAT:	7.1G
CARBOHYDRATES:	14.8G
TOTAL SUGAR:	1.9G
FIBRE:	3.5G
SODIUM:	2.2G

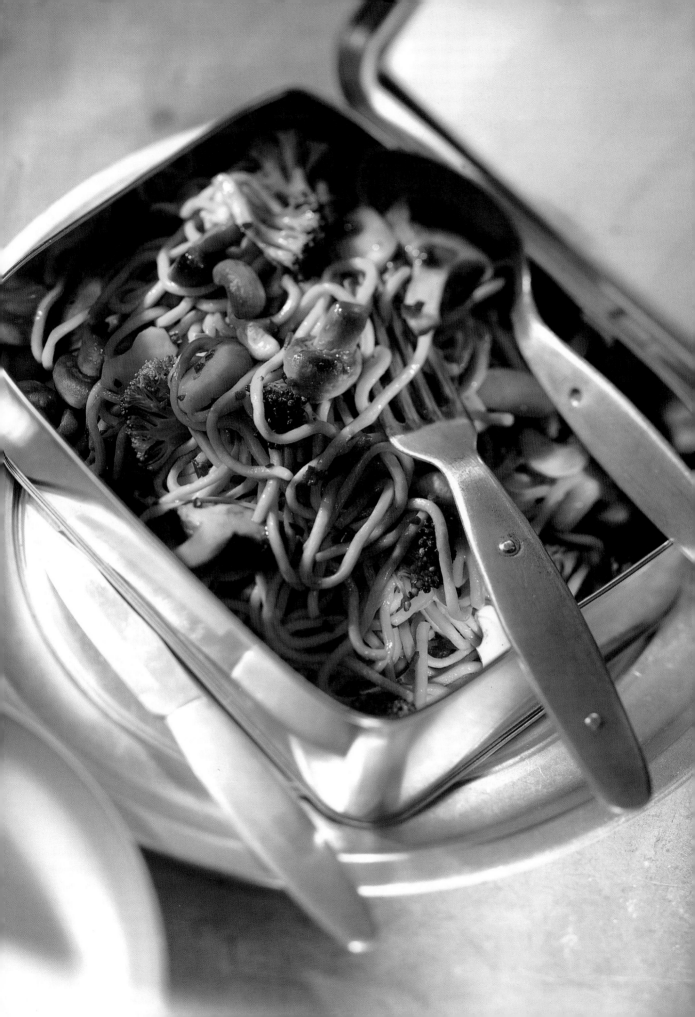

Tofu-filled wontons
with mushrooms and peppers in yellow bean sauce

SERVES 4 AS A MAIN COURSE, 6 AS A STARTER

INGREDIENTS

275 g/10 oz **tofu**

½ teaspoon **bouillon powder**

1 tablespoon **sunflower oil**

1 small **leek** or 2–3 spring onions, finely sliced

100 g/3½ oz shiitake **mushrooms**, finely sliced

1 tablespoon **tamari**

1 **garlic clove**, crushed

dash of **Tabasco** sauce

1 teaspoon **sesame seeds**, toasted

24 **wonton skins** (8 x 6 cm/3 x 2½ inches)

small bunch of **coriander**

YELLOW BEAN SAUCE

1 very small **leek** or 2 spring onions, finely sliced

1 tablespoon **sunflower oil**

100 g/3½ oz shiitake **mushrooms**, finely sliced

1 **garlic clove**, crushed

125 g/4 oz **yellow bean** sauce

2 cm/¾ inch piece of fresh **ginger**, grated

1 cm/½ inch piece of fresh **chilli**, finely chopped

¼ **red** and ¼ **green pepper**, finely diced

NUTRITIONAL INFORMATION
one serving contains

CALORIES:	383
TOTAL FAT:	12.7 G
CARBOHYDRATES:	54.7 G
TOTAL SUGAR:	7.3 G
FIBRE:	3.3 G
SODIUM:	2.9 G

These are a little fiddly to make, and you must endeavour to stick the sides together as best they will, but they are truly worth the effort.

METHOD

1. For the tofu filling, crumble the tofu and sprinkle with the bouillon powder. Heat the sunflower oil and sauté the leek or spring onions for 1–2 minutes, then add the mushrooms, tamari and garlic and sauté until the mushrooms are beginning to soften. Add the tofu and cook for a further 1–2 minutes, adding a dash of Tabasco and a splash of water to prevent sticking. Add the sesame seeds and remove from the heat.

2. Place the wonton skins flat on the work surface and add 2 teaspoons of filling to each. Moisten the edges and seal to make four-pointed parcels.

3. For the sauce, sauté the leek or spring onions in the oil, then add the mushrooms and garlic and cook until softened. Add the yellow bean sauce and 3 tablespoons water, then squeeze in the juice from the ginger, the chopped chilli and diced peppers. Stir and remove from the heat.

4. The wontons can be steamed or poached in gently simmering water for 2–3 minutes until translucent. Serve with the sauce, with the coriander scattered over.

Stir-fried green pepper
and shiitake mushrooms with roasted courgettes and tofu

SERVES 4

INGREDIENTS

275 g/10 oz **tofu**, cut into chunks

6 tablespoons **tamari**

1 **garlic clove**, crushed

dash of **Tabasco** sauce, or a small piece of chilli, finely diced

2 **courgettes**, cut into large chunks

2½ teaspoons **sunflower oil**

350 g/13 oz packet of **udon noodles** (or egg noodles)

2 **green peppers**, cut into large chunks

250 g/9 oz shiitake **mushrooms**, sliced

3 cm/1 inch piece of fresh **ginger**, grated

125 g/4 oz **black bean** sauce

1 teaspoon **tamarind paste**

Roasting the courgettes in this way gives them a melting texture that is quite unexpected in a stir-fry dish,

METHOD

1. Marinate the tofu in the tamari mixed with the garlic, Tabasco and 6 tablespoons water for at least 1 hour. Preheat the oven to 220°C/425°F/gas 7.

2. Mix the courgettes with 1 teaspoon of the oil and place in an ovenproof dish. Drain the tofu, add to the courgettes and roast for about 20 minutes, until both courgettes and tofu are golden brown.

3. Cook the noodles according to the packet instructions.

4. Heat the remaining 1½ teaspoons oil in a wok and fry the peppers over a high heat until the skins start to blister. Add the mushrooms and continue to cook for about 1 minute or until the mushrooms soften, adding a little water if they begin to stick.

5. Squeeze the juice from the ginger into the wok. Add the black bean sauce and tamarind paste, the chopped chilli if using, stir through and serve at once on a bed of noodles, topped with the roasted tofu and courgettes.

NUTRITIONAL INFORMATION
one serving contains

CALORIES:	505
TOTAL FAT:	14.6 G
CARBOHYDRATES:	74.3 G
TOTAL SUGAR:	9.8 G
FIBRE:	5.5 G
SODIUM:	6.1 G

Celeriac casserole in cabbage leaves

SERVES 6

INGREDIENTS

1 Savoy **cabbage**

3 tablespoons **olive oil**

1 small **red onion**, finely chopped

2 **garlic cloves**, crushed

3 teaspoons **garam masala**

½ teaspoon ground **coriander**

2 teaspoons **paprika**

750 g/1 lb 10 oz **potatoes**, peeled and diced

750 g/1 lb 10 oz **celeriac**, peeled, cut into 1 cm/
  ½ inch thick slices, then diced

salt and pepper

250 g/9 oz chestnut (or button) **mushrooms**,
  quartered

1 tablespoon **tamari**

juice of 1 small **lemon**

50 g/2 oz **green beans**, blanched and diced, or
  spinach, shredded

½ **red pepper**, very finely diced

1 teaspoon **harissa** or other chilli sauce

a good handful of fresh **parsley**, chopped

NUTRITIONAL INFORMATION one serving contains	
CALORIES:	240
TOTAL FAT:	9.7 G
CARBOHYDRATES:	32 G
TOTAL SUGAR:	7.9 G
FIBRE:	9.9 G
SODIUM:	0.9 G

A hearty, satisfying casserole to warm you on a winter's day.

METHOD

1. Separate six outer leaves from the cabbage and blanch in boiling water for 1 minute. Drain and refresh in cold water. Set aside.

2. Halve or quarter the remaining cabbage (depending on size), cut out the core and cut a piece weighing about 100 g/3½ oz. Shred with a long, sharp knife.

3. Heat 2½ tablespoons of the oil in a large saucepan, add the onion and garlic and fry until translucent. Add the garam masala, coriander and paprika and fry for 1–2 minutes, adding 2–3 tablespoons of water to loosen the spices.

4. Add the potatoes and stir over the heat for 2–3 minutes. Add the celeriac, salt and pepper and keep stirring over a low heat, adding 2–3 tablespoons of water from time to time to prevent sticking.

5. Heat 1 teaspoon of the oil in a saucepan and sauté the mushrooms for 2–3 minutes, adding the tamari and a little water. Add the sautéed mushrooms and shredded cabbage to the casserole and continue to stir over the heat, adding a little water from time to time – you will need to add about 250 ml/8 fl oz water in total. After 25–30 minutes, the potatoes and celeriac should be tender but not falling apart.

6. To serve, add the lemon juice, then the beans, red pepper and harissa. Spoon generously into the blanched outer leaves of the cabbage. Garnish with plenty of chopped parsley and pour over any remaining liquid from the pan. Serve hot.

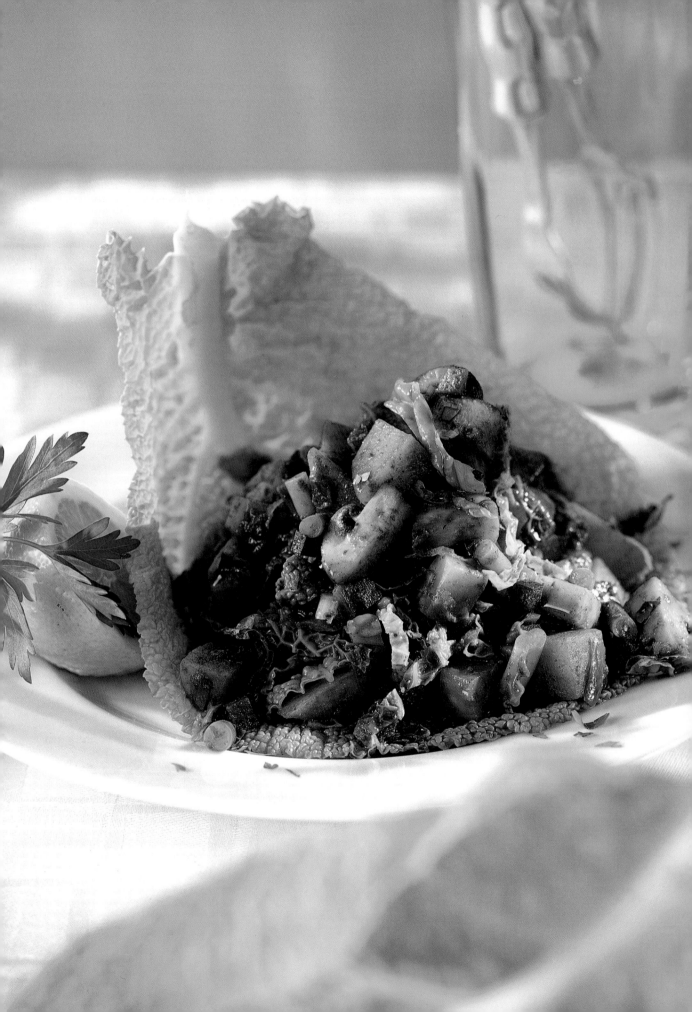

Cannellini bean casserole
with spinach and smoked tofu

SERVES 4–6

INGREDIENTS
1 **red pepper**

2 tablespoons **olive oil**

200 g/7 oz **smoked tofu**, cut into matchsticks

2 tablespoons **tamari**

100 g/3½ oz **mushrooms**, sliced

1 tablespoon **red wine** (optional)

3 x 400 g/14 oz cans of **cannellini beans**
   (including the liquid)

dash of **Tabasco** sauce

freshly grated **nutmeg**

freshly ground black pepper

1 teaspoon **wholegrain mustard**

200 g/7 oz fresh **spinach**

This is a mercifully quick winter stew. Use a good olive oil for flavour. Allow the stew to stand for a while and mash some of the beans before eating. The red pepper and spinach provide vitamin A and iron, and there'll be even more if you garnish with extra chopped parsley.

METHOD
1. Preheat the grill to very hot. Grill the pepper until the skin begins to blacken. Leave to cool slightly, then peel, cut into strips and set aside.
2. Heat 1 tablespoon of the oil in a wide saucepan, add the tofu and sauté, turning frequently, for about 1 minute. Add half the tamari and continue to sauté until the tofu begins to become brown and crisp, stirring frequently, without letting the tofu break up. Remove from the pan and set aside.
3. Heat the remaining oil in the pan and add the mushrooms, remaining tamari and red wine, if using. Sauté for 2–3 minutes, then remove and set aside.
4. Empty the contents of the three cans of beans into the pan. Add a dash of Tabasco, nutmeg, pepper and the mustard. Simmer for 5–6 minutes, stirring frequently and allowing some of the beans to break up slightly. Add the spinach and continue to cook for 2–3 minutes, then add the mushrooms and red pepper strips and heat through for a further 2–3 minutes. Serve hot, with some of the crisp smoked tofu scattered over the vegetables.

NUTRITIONAL INFORMATION
one serving contains

CALORIES:	430
TOTAL FAT:	12.1G
CARBOHYDRATES:	56.7G
TOTAL SUGAR:	6.5G
FIBRE:	20.5G
SODIUM:	1.5G

Fennel and mushroom casserole

SERVES 6

INGREDIENTS

3 tablespoons **olive oil**

2 small **red onions**, cut into 8 wedges

½ teaspoon dried **marjoram**

2 **garlic cloves**, sliced

sea salt and coarsely ground black pepper

800 g/1¾ lb **fennel** (preferably small young
   bulbs), trimmed, reserving fronds, then cut
   lengthways into chunks

2 teaspoons **bouillon powder** dissolved in
   200 ml/7 fl oz water

750 g/1 lb 10 oz chestnut (or button)
   mushrooms, cleaned and quartered

6–7 drops of **Tabasco** sauce

1 teaspoon **wholegrain mustard**

1 teaspoon **lemon juice**

2 teaspoons **cornflour** dissolved in
   2 teaspoons water

700 g/1½ lb baby **spinach**

2 **tomatoes**, de-seeded and diced

4 small sprigs of **basil**

boiled brown **rice**, new potatoes or pasta,
   to serve

**Apart from the oil, this is incredibly low in fat.
Serve it with rice, new potatoes boiled in their
skins, or big, fat pappardelle noodles.**

METHOD

1. Heat the oil in a large saucepan and add the onions, marjoram, garlic, and a good pinch of salt and pepper. Sauté until the onion is translucent.

2. Add the fennel and bouillon. Cover and bring to the boil, then reduce the heat and simmer for 10 minutes.

3. Add the mushrooms and simmer for a further 7–8 minutes, stirring occasionally.

4. Add the Tabasco, mustard and lemon juice, then the dissolved cornflour. Just before serving, stir in the spinach and garnish with the diced tomatoes and basil. Serve hot, with rice, potatoes or pasta.

NUTRITIONAL INFORMATION one serving contains	
CALORIES:	333
TOTAL FAT:	11.3 G
CARBOHYDRATES:	50 G
TOTAL SUGAR:	7.3 G
FIBRE:	8.8 G
SODIUM:	1.4 G

Vegetable brochettes

SERVES 6

INGREDIENTS

24 large button **mushrooms**

3 **red peppers**, cut into quarters

3 **courgettes**, scored along the length with a
fork and cut into 2 cm/¾ inch pieces

1 large **aubergine**, cut into 12 slices

175 g/6 oz **haloumi** cheese, cut into 3 cm x
1 cm/1 x ½ inch pieces

juice of 1 **lime**

2 tablespoons **extra-virgin olive oil**

dash of **Tabasco** sauce

15 g/½ oz fresh **coriander**

1 heaped tablespoon finely chopped **pistachios**

couscous or couscous salad (page 102),
to serve

MARINADE

1 tablespoon **cumin**

1 tablespoon **paprika**

3 tablespoons **tamari**

1½ tablespoons **olive oil**

2 **garlic cloves**, crushed

dash of **Tabasco** sauce

NUTRITIONAL INFORMATION one serving contains	
CALORIES:	572
TOTAL FAT:	24 G
CARBOHYDRATES:	72.4 G
TOTAL SUGAR:	15 G
FIBRE:	5.6 G
SODIUM:	2.6 G

The salty haloumi cheese makes this perfect for summer, but if you are anxious about the fat content, substitute a half-fat mozzarella. Take care, though – it will melt very quickly and needs no pre-grilling. Serve as part of a Middle Eastern-style mezze with several salads, bowls of olives and warmed pitta bread.

METHOD

1. Combine all the marinade ingredients in a large shallow dish, add 3 tablespoons water and a pinch of salt and mix well. Add the mushrooms, pepper pieces and courgette pieces and marinate for at least 1 hour. Soak twelve 15 cm/6 inch wooden satay sticks in cold water.

2. Meanwhile, lightly baste the aubergine slices with the same marinade but keep them apart from the other vegetables. Cook the aubergine under a preheated grill for 3–4 minutes until golden brown, turning once to brown evenly.

3. Lay the pieces of haloumi on a lightly oiled baking sheet and grill for a couple of minutes, until golden brown but not melting. Wrap the aubergine slices around the pieces of haloumi.

4. Skewer the marinated vegetables on to the satay sticks, beginning and ending with a mushroom. Put the brochettes on a baking sheet and place under a hot grill for a few minutes, turning to ensure that they are well grilled on all sides. Remove from the heat.

5. Mix the olive oil, Tabasco, lime juice and coriander and drizzle over the vegetables. Finally sprinkle with the finely chopped pistachios and serve at once, with couscous.

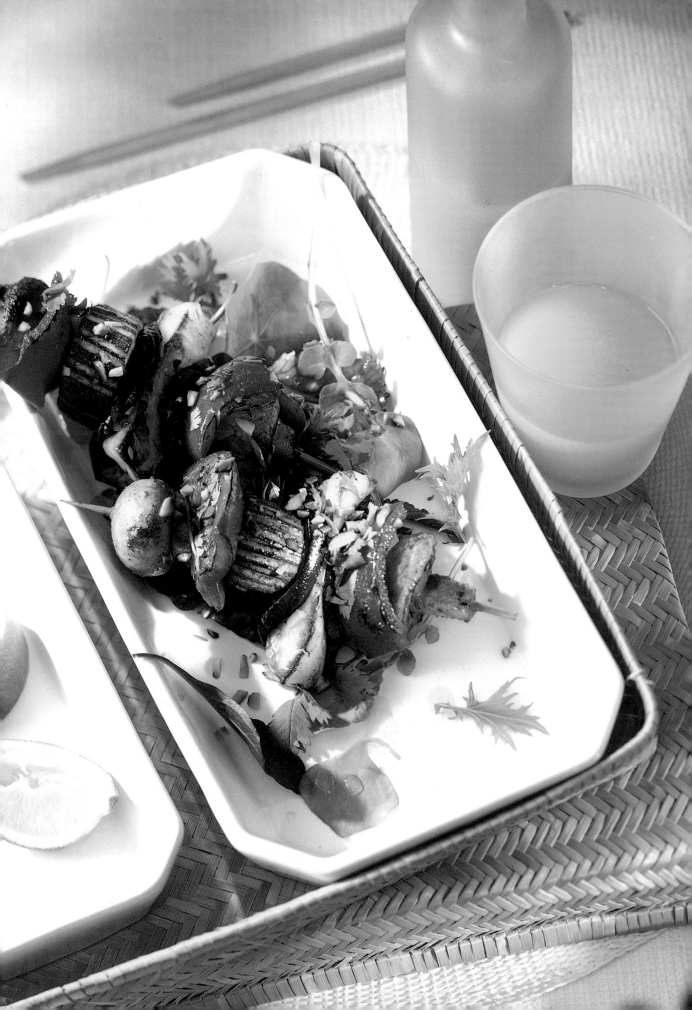

Light lasagne

SERVES 8

INGREDIENTS

2 large **courgettes**, cut into chunks

1 tablespoon **olive oil**

salt and freshly ground black pepper

300 g/11 oz **mushrooms**, halved or quartered

1 teaspoon **tamari**

250 g/9 oz fresh **spinach**

1 large **red pepper**

375 g/13 oz low-fat **fromage frais**

400 g/14 oz 98% fat-free **bio yoghurt**

½ teaspoon **bouillon powder**

1 **garlic clove**, crushed

200 g/7 oz fresh **pasta sheets**

TOMATO SAUCE

1 kg/2¼ lb (2½ cans) canned chopped **tomatoes**

1 small **red onion**, finely chopped

3 **garlic cloves**, crushed

1 tablespoon **olive oil**

25 g/1 oz **tomato purée**

25 g/1 oz **black olives**, cut into slivers

small handful of fresh **basil**

½ teaspoon **Tabasco** sauce

NUTRITIONAL INFORMATION one serving contains	
CALORIES:	224
TOTAL FAT:	6G
CARBOHYDRATES:	31.5G
TOTAL SUGAR:	15.1G
FIBRE:	3.8G
SODIUM:	1.1G

This recipe avoids the heavy, cloying feeling of a conventional lasagne.

METHOD

1. First make the tomato sauce. Put all the ingredients into a saucepan, bring to the boil, then reduce the heat and simmer until thick, about 25 minutes. Season to taste.

2. Preheat the oven to 220°C/425°F/gas 7. Put the courgettes into an ovenproof dish with the oil, 1 tablespoon water, salt and pepper. Roast for 10–12 minutes, or until golden brown, then add to the tomato sauce.

3. Sauté the mushrooms with the tamari and a little salt and pepper; they will release and cook in their own juice. Add to the tomato sauce.

4. Wash the spinach and place in a saucepan with a pinch of salt and pepper. Place over a medium heat for a minute or two, until the spinach wilts.

5. Cut eight 1 cm/½ inch strips of red pepper and set aside. Chop the remaining red pepper into large pieces and add to the tomato sauce.

6. Mix together the fromage frais, yoghurt, bouillon powder and garlic. Add half this mixture to the spinach and stir to mix.

7. To assemble the lasagne: pour one-third of the tomato and vegetable sauce into a 28 x 18 cm/ 11 x 7 inch ovenproof dish. Add a layer of pasta, then another one-third of the tomato sauce. Add the cheese, yoghurt and spinach mixture and cover with pasta. Top with the remaining tomato sauce, then the plain cheese mixture. Arrange the strips of red pepper on top to mark the centre of each portion. Bake in the oven for about 30 minutes. Serve hot.

Broccoli booster

SERVES 6

INGREDIENTS

2 **red peppers**

3 tablespoons **olive oil**

1 small **red onion**, roughly chopped

1 litre/1¾ pints chopped **tomatoes**

1 teaspoon **tomato purée**

3 **garlic cloves**, finely sliced

½ teaspoon **sugar**

salt and pepper

large handful of fresh **basil**

500 g/1 lb 2 oz **broccoli** florets

500 g/1 lb 2 oz **courgettes**, cut into chunks

50 g/2 oz **mushrooms**, sliced

1 teaspoon **cornflour** dissolved in 1 teaspoon
  water (optional)

200 g/7 oz cooked (or canned) **butter beans**

4 **tomatoes**, cut into 4 or 6 wedges, depending
  on size

dash of **Tabasco** sauce

boiled brown **rice**, to serve

Everything depends on the freshness and crisp-ness of the vegetables, and on the dish being eaten when freshly made. Old-fashioned vegetarian food, but a good standby for days when you need something childishly simple. Packed with vitamins, hence its name, this could be made healthier still by pairing it with a bowl of steaming brown rice.

METHOD

1. Preheat the grill to very hot. Grill the peppers until the skins begin to blacken. Leave to cool slightly, then peel, cut into strips and set aside.

2. Heat the oil, add the onion and fry until translucent. Add the chopped tomatoes, tomato purée, garlic, sugar, salt, pepper and half the basil. Bring to the boil, then reduce the heat and simmer for about 20 minutes.

3. Meanwhile, cook the broccoli in boiling salted water for 2 minutes. Drain, reserving the water, and refresh the broccoli in cold water. Bring the water back to the boil, add the courgettes and boil for 20–30 seconds.

4. Add the mushrooms to the tomato sauce and simmer for about 2 minutes, then stir in the dissolved cornflour, if using, the red pepper strips, broccoli, courgettes, butter beans and tomato wedges. Heat through, adding a dash of Tabasco sauce and adjusting the seasoning if necessary. Garnish with basil and serve hot, with brown rice.

NUTRITIONAL INFORMATION one serving contains	
CALORIES:	383
TOTAL FAT:	10.8 G
CARBOHYDRATES:	61.1 G
TOTAL SUGAR:	15.3 G
FIBRE:	8.6 G
SODIUM:	0.7 G

Five roasted roots
with a tikka spice sauce

SERVES 6

INGREDIENTS

6 tablespoons **tikka paste**

2 tablespoons **olive oil**

2 tablespoons **pineapple juice**

1 teaspoon **cornflour** (optional)

650 g/1 lb 6 oz low-fat **bio yoghurt**

500 g/1 lb 2 oz **beetroot**, cut into 2 cm/¾ inch cubes – or left whole if you can get baby beetroot

500 g/1 lb 2 oz **carrots**, cut into 1 cm/½ inch thick slices

500 g/1 lb 2 oz **parsnips**, cut into 1 cm/½ inch thick slices

500 g/1 lb 2 oz **potatoes**, cut into 2 cm/¾ inch cubes

500 g/1 lb 2 oz **sweet potatoes**, cut into 2 cm/¾ inch cubes

small handful of fresh **rosemary**

small handful of fresh **thyme**

1 teaspoon **garam masala**

salt and freshly ground black pepper

large handful of fresh **parsley**, finely chopped

The complexities and depth of flavour in Indian seasonings lend themselves brilliantly to hybridization. This is one recipe in that direction.

METHOD

1. Heat the oven to 200°C/400°F/gas 6.
2. Mix 2 tablespoons of the tikka paste with the oil, pineapple juice and cornflour, if using, then mix with 250 g/9 oz of the yoghurt. Keeping the beetroot and sweet potatoes separate, coat all the vegetables in the yoghurt mixture.
3. Spread the beetroot on a baking sheet and place in the hot oven. After 5 minutes, add the carrots, parsnips and potatoes. After a further 5 minutes, add the sweet potatoes. Bake for a further 35 minutes, or until the vegetables are tender but still firm.
4. Transfer all the vegetables to a large saucepan and add the rosemary, thyme and remaining yoghurt. Simmer for 5–10 minutes, adding more yoghurt if necessary. Season with garam masala, salt and pepper, sprinkle with the chopped parsley and serve at once.

NUTRITIONAL INFORMATION
one serving contains

CALORIES:	393
TOTAL FAT:	11.2 G
CARBOHYDRATES:	64.4 G
TOTAL SUGAR:	29.6 G
FIBRE:	10.6 G
SODIUM:	1.3 G

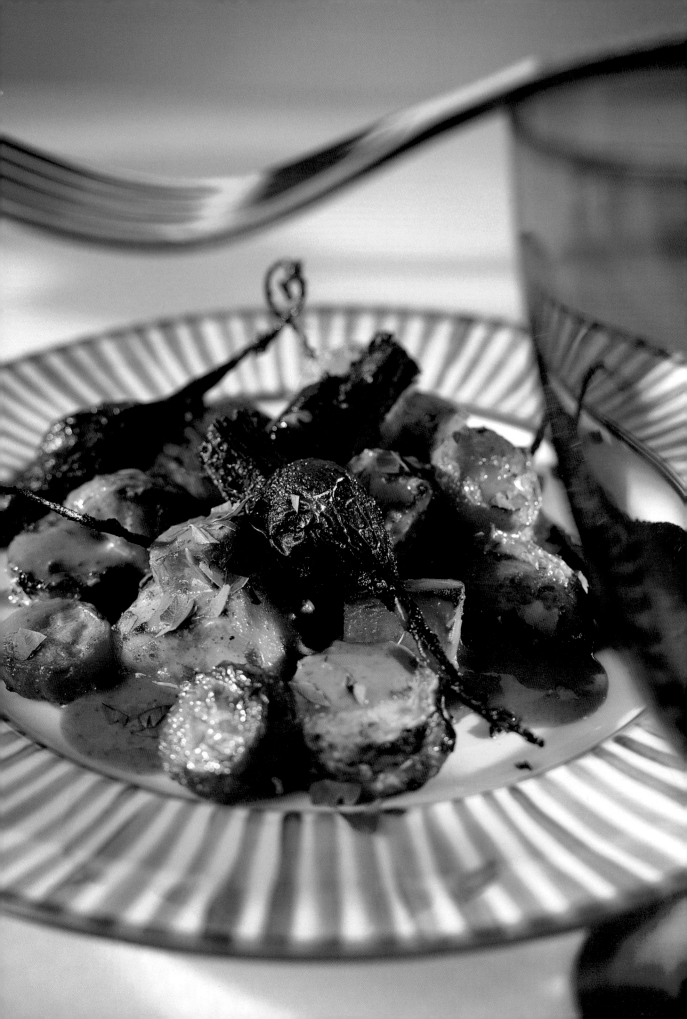

Spinach and ricotta gnocchi
in roasted tomato broth

SERVES 6

INGREDIENTS

600 g/1¼ lb fresh **spinach** (or 350 g/13 oz
 frozen)

salt and pepper

freshly grated **nutmeg**

1 **garlic clove**, crushed

225 g/8 oz **ricotta**

85 g/3 oz plain **flour**

25 g/1 oz **Parmesan** cheese, grated

ROASTED TOMATO BROTH

750 g/1 lb 10 oz **vine-ripened tomatoes**,
 cut in half

sea salt and cracked black pepper

2 **garlic cloves**, chopped

2 tablespoons **olive oil**

TO SERVE

sprigs of **basil**

grated **Parmesan** cheese, (optional)

cracked black pepper

French bread or **ciabatta**

NUTRITIONAL INFORMATION one serving contains	
CALORIES:	361
TOTAL FAT:	13.4 G
CARBOHYDRATES:	47.7 G
TOTAL SUGAR:	7.4 G
FIBRE:	4.7 G
SODIUM:	1.7 G

I urge you to develop a passion for these. Much easier to make than they sound, they will stand you in good stead and everyone is always impressed. Serve with warmed French bread or ciabatta to mop up the tomato broth.

METHOD

1. First make the tomato broth. Preheat the oven to 200°C/400°F/gas 6. Place the tomato halves on a baking sheet and sprinkle with the salt and pepper, garlic and oil. Roast in the oven for about 40 minutes, then blend until smooth. For a really smooth result, rub through a sieve.

2. Wash the fresh spinach and place in a saucepan over medium heat. When the spinach has wilted, drain well and chop finely. (If using frozen spinach, heat through, then drain and chop.) Mix in the salt, pepper, nutmeg and garlic, then stir in the ricotta, flour and Parmesan. Form into walnut-sized balls.

3. Bring a large saucepan of salted water to the boil, then reduce to a simmer. Add some of the gnocchi and simmer for about 2 minutes, or until they rise to the surface. Lift one out to test that it is cooked and no longer floury. Lift out the cooked gnocchi, using a slotted spoon, and keep warm while you cook the rest.

4. Reheat the tomato broth and serve in six large flat soup plates. Place six gnocchi in each plate and garnish with basil, Parmesan and black pepper. Serve with warmed bread.

Sweet potato gnocchi
with rocket sauce

SERVES 4

INGREDIENTS

1 kg/2¼ lb **sweet potatoes**

100 g/3½ oz plain **flour**

pinch of grated **nutmeg**

salt and pepper

1 **red onion**, finely diced

ROCKET SAUCE

2 tablespoons **olive oil**

1 **spring onion**, finely sliced

½ teaspoon fresh **lemon juice**

1 teaspoon **tamari**

40 g/1½ oz **rocket**, finely shredded

25 g/1 oz **Pecorino** cheese (or Parmesan)

As with the spinach gnocchi, these are not difficult to make. Just make sure that the 'dough' is not too wet – which is why the potatoes must be baked, not boiled. Try one out first: if it falls apart, add a little more flour. On the other hand, too much flour will make them sticky. With a little experimentation, you will soon develop a feel for them.

METHOD

1. Preheat the oven to 250°C/475°F/gas 8. Bake the potatoes in their skins until tender, about 40 minutes, depending on size. Scoop out the flesh and mash with the flour, nutmeg and salt and pepper to taste. Mix in the diced onion, then shape into quenelles, using about 2 teaspoons of the mixture for each quenelle.

2. Bring a large saucepan of water to the boil, then reduce to a simmer. Drop in the quenelles and simmer until they rise to the surface – you will need to do this in several batches. Drain and keep warm.

3. Mix together all the ingredients for the sauce. Serve the gnocchi as soon as they are all done, with the sauce poured over them.

NUTRITIONAL INFORMATION one serving contains	
CALORIES:	410
TOTAL FAT:	10.8 G
CARBOHYDRATES:	75 G
TOTAL SUGAR:	16.3 G
FIBRE:	7.3 G
SODIUM:	0.9 G

Butternut squash parcels
with wild mushrooms, red onions and garlic

SERVES 4

INGREDIENTS

2 **butternut squash**

175 g/6 oz chanterelle **mushrooms**,
   cleaned of grit

2 small **red onions**, cut into 6 or 8, depending
   on size

2 tablespoons **tamari**

1 tablespoon **red wine** or **marsala**

dash of **Tabasco** sauce

2 tablespoons **olive oil**

4 small sprigs of **rosemary**

1 whole head of **garlic**, separated into cloves

8–10 blanched **almonds**, cut in half

rice or couscous, to serve

Although by no means difficult to do, this is one of those dishes that makes a great impression at the table, as the paper or foil parcels are opened to release a cloud of fragrant steam. A mixture of brown and wild rice would be my accompaniment of choice.

METHOD

1. Preheat the oven to 200°C/400°F/gas 6. Cut out four squares of baking parchment (or kitchen foil), 25 x 25 cm/10 x 10 inches.

2. Cut each squash in half, remove the seeds and cut the flesh into 3 cm/1 inch chunks. Place in a large bowl and add the mushrooms and onions.

3. Mix the tamari, red wine, Tabasco and olive oil with 1 tablespoon water. Mix with the vegetables and the remaining ingredients. Divide the mixture between the squares of baking parchment, making sure each parcel has a couple of cloves of garlic, a sprig of rosemary and at least two almonds. Fold and pinch the edges of the paper together to seal the parcels, then place in the oven for 25 minutes. Serve at once, accompanied by rice or couscous.

NUTRITIONAL INFORMATION
one serving contains

CALORIES:	435
TOTAL FAT:	10.3 G
CARBOHYDRATES:	79.3 G
TOTAL SUGAR:	20.6 G
FIBRE:	8.5 G
SODIUM:	1.2 G

Pasta with mushrooms and brandy

SERVES 4–6

INGREDIENTS

250 g/9 oz **pasta** (not made with eggs)

250 g/9 oz button **mushrooms**

bunch of **tarragon**, leaves stripped and roughly chopped

4 **garlic cloves**, crushed

4 tablespoons **tamari**

2 tablespoons **brandy**

2 tablespoons **olive oil**

dash of **Tabasco** sauce

250 g/9 oz mixed **wild mushrooms** (oyster, chanterelle, shiitake), sliced thickly

1 teaspoon **cornflour** dissolved in 1 tablespoon water

When they are all used together, nothing concentrates the flavours of mushrooms quite like garlic, tamari and brandy. You will never miss the cream in this perfect alternative to the ubiquitous pasta al funghi.

METHOD

1. Preheat the grill to high. Cook the pasta in plenty of boiling water.
2. Put the button mushrooms, tarragon, garlic, tamari, brandy, oil and Tabasco in a frying pan and sauté over a gentle heat for 3–4 minutes, until the mushrooms have released their juices.
3. Meanwhile, baste the wild mushrooms with 3 tablespoons of the tarragon and tamari liquid, then grill until they are just cooked.
4. Add the dissolved cornflour to the button mushrooms and cook, stirring, for 1–2 minutes to thicken.
5. Add the grilled mushrooms to the button mushrooms, toss with the drained cooked pasta and serve at once.

NUTRITIONAL INFORMATION one serving contains	
CALORIES:	337
TOTAL FAT:	9.2 G
CARBOHYDRATES:	51.5 G
TOTAL SUGAR:	1.6 G
FIBRE:	2.8 G
SODIUM:	2.3 G

Filled tomatoes
with cannellini beans

SERVES 6

INGREDIENTS

3 slices of **wholemeal bread**, cubed

6 large **beef tomatoes**

2 x 400 g/14 oz cans of **cannellini beans**,
  drained

450 g/1 lb **broad beans**, blanched and peeled

2 **red onions**, finely diced

10 **black olives**, roughly chopped

bunch of **basil**

2 **garlic cloves**, crushed

1½ teaspoons **tamari**

1½ teaspoons **balsamic vinegar**

1 teaspoon **Tabasco** sauce

salt and pepper

3 tablespoons **olive oil**

Serve these with basmati rice or couscous, or serve the tomatoes on their own as a first course.

METHOD

1. Preheat the oven to 180°C/350°F/gas 4. Lightly toast the bread cubes in the oven, then set aside.

2. Slice the tomatoes in half and scoop the seeds and flesh into a sieve. Leave the tomato halves upside down to drain. Rub the flesh through the sieve over a bowl to catch the juice.

3. Mix the cannellini and broad beans with the tomato juice, onions, olives, basil leaves, garlic, tamari, vinegar, Tabasco, salt and pepper. Spoon this mixture into the tomato halves, reserving any that won't fit in. Place the tomatoes on a baking sheet, drizzle with olive oil and bake for 15 minutes.

4. Add the croûtons to the tomatoes and return to the oven for 5 minutes. Warm any remaining bean mixture in a saucepan and pour over the tomatoes just before serving.

NUTRITIONAL INFORMATION one serving contains	
CALORIES:	283
TOTAL FAT:	10.4 G
CARBOHYDRATES:	36.4 G
TOTAL SUGAR:	10.4 G
FIBRE:	12.45 G
SODIUM:	1.7 G

Roasted butternut squash
with coconut and coriander sauce

SERVES 6

INGREDIENTS

3 **butternut squash**, about 700 g/1½ lb each

1½ tablespoons **olive oil**

1 teaspoon **tamari**

2 dashes of **Tabasco** sauce

few drops of **balsamic vinegar**

1 **garlic clove**, crushed

COCONUT AND CORIANDER SAUCE

400 ml/14 fl oz canned **coconut milk**

1 **garlic clove**, sliced

1 **spring onion**, sliced

¼ **red pepper**, finely diced

large handful of fresh **coriander**

salt and pepper

Some coconut milk is thicker than others; leaving the sauce to stand gives it a chance to thicken up, but it doesn't matter if it seems thin – it will be absorbed by the squash. Basmati rice would be a happy accompaniment.

METHOD

1. Heat the oven to 200°C/400°F/gas 6. Cut the squash in half lengthways and remove the seeds. Make deep cuts in the flesh – but not all the way through to the skin – to form a diamond pattern.

2. Mix the oil, tamari and Tabasco, vinegar and garlic together with ½ tablespoon water and brush over the squash. Turn the squash flesh side down on a baking sheet and bake for 35–40 minutes, until the flesh is tender. Turn the squash flesh side up and bake for a further 10 minutes.

3. Meanwhile, make the sauce. Put the coconut milk, garlic, spring onion, half the red pepper and half the coriander into a saucepan, simmer for 10 minutes, then turn off the heat and leave to infuse.

4. To serve, strain the sauce and return to the pan to reheat. Add the remaining red pepper and coriander and salt to taste. Spoon a little over each squash and serve the rest separately.

NUTRITIONAL INFORMATION one serving contains	
CALORIES:	182
TOTAL FAT:	4.4 G
CARBOHYDRATES:	33.4 G
TOTAL SUGAR:	19.6 G
FIBRE:	5.8 G
SODIUM:	0.8 G

COUSCOUS

It's taken years and years but **couscous** is finally here to stay – and all because someone realized that you could reconstitute it in a matter of minutes by **simply** pouring boiling water or stock over it, instead of steaming it for hours in a couscousier. And someone else realized that it's low in fat and that it makes you feel incredibly full but that it's **easily** digested. Now it's as much a staple as pasta or rice. It can be eaten hot or cold and **loves** all manner of vegetables, especially served with spicy harissa and a bowl of strong broth on the side.

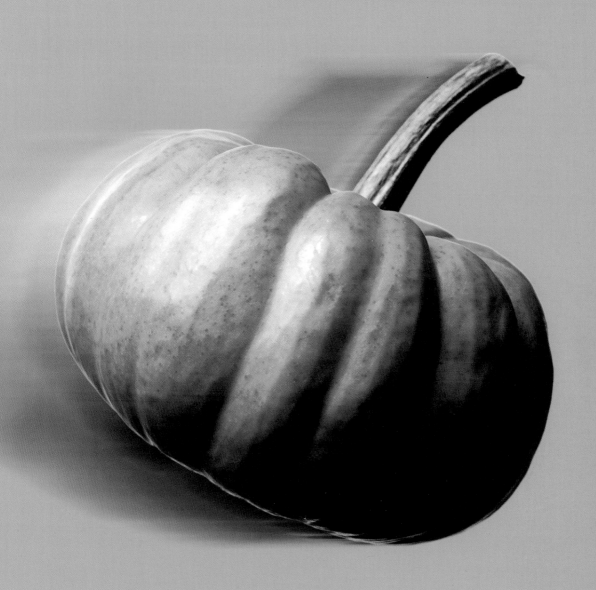

Basic couscous

SERVES 6–8

INGREDIENTS

500 g/1 lb 2 oz **couscous**

2 teaspoons **bouillon powder** (optional)

2 tablespoons chopped fresh **coriander**

1 tablespoon **wholegrain mustard**

1 teaspoon **lemon juice**

salt and pepper

This is my tried and tested way of packing maximum flavour into couscous.

METHOD

1. Put the couscous in a bowl and add enough boiling water to cover the couscous by about 1 cm/½ inch (or follow the packet instructions). Leave to stand until the couscous is soft, about 10 minutes.

2. Add all the remaining ingredients and mix well, using a fork to separate the grains of couscous. If you like, accompany with yoghurt, yoghurt sauce or harissa.

COUSCOUS SALAD

To the basic couscous (above), add 2 tomatoes, ½ red pepper and ½ cucumber – all diced – together with the juice of 1 lemon and 2 tablespoons raisins.

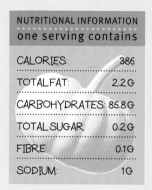

NUTRITIONAL INFORMATION
one serving contains

CALORIES:	386
TOTAL FAT:	2.2 G
CARBOHYDRATES:	85.8 G
TOTAL SUGAR:	0.2 G
FIBRE:	0.1 G
SODIUM:	1 G

Curried parsnip couscous
with mango relish

INGREDIENTS

750 g/1 lb 10 oz **parsnips**, peeled and trimmed

1 teaspoon **paprika**

1 teaspoon ground **cumin**

1 tablespoon **honey**

1 teaspoon sea salt

dash of **Tabasco** sauce

1 tablespoon **sunflower oil**

Basic **couscous** (see page 102)

handful of fresh **coriander leaves**

MANGO RELISH

1 ripe, firm **mango**, cut into small dice

2 tablespoons chopped fresh **coriander**

½ **red onion**, very finely chopped

1 fresh **chilli,** very finely chopped

Use young, small parsnips if you can. Blanching them briefly would reduce the required roasting time, and you may prefer to do this because the parsnips must be crisp on the outside and very soft in the middle.

METHOD

1. Cut the parsnips into 7 cm/3 inch batons (they should be about 1.5 cm/⅝ inch in diameter, so you may need to halve or quarter them lengthways).

2. Mix the paprika, cumin, honey, salt, Tabasco and oil together, pour over the parsnips and leave to marinate for 30 minutes.

3. Preheat the oven to 200°C/400°F/gas 6. Cover the parsnips tightly with foil and bake for 45 minutes to 1 hour. Turn them regularly, making sure they are tightly wrapped when you return them to the oven. You may need to sprinkle them with water from time to time to prevent sticking.

4. Towards the end of the roasting time, prepare the couscous.

5. Mix all the ingredients for the mango relish and warm through. Serve with the couscous and parsnips, sprinkled with fresh coriander leaves.

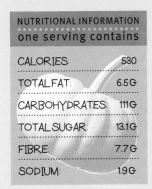

NUTRITIONAL INFORMATION one serving contains	
CALORIES	530
TOTAL FAT	6.5G
CARBOHYDRATES	111G
TOTAL SUGAR	13.1G
FIBRE	7.7G
SODIUM	1.9G

Moroccan vegetable couscous

SERVES 6–8

INGREDIENTS

1 kg/2¼ lb **pumpkin** (weight with seeds removed), cut into 4 cm/1½ inch chunks

1 small **white cabbage**, cut into 4 cm/1½ inch chunks

300 g/11 oz **carrots**, cut into 5 cm/2 inch pieces

3 thin **leeks**, cut into 5 cm/2 inch lengths

300 g/11 oz **parsnips**, halved or quartered lengthways, then cut into 5 cm/2 inch pieces

300 g/11 oz **courgettes**, halved or quartered lengthways, then cut into 5 cm/2 inch pieces

500 g/1 lb 2 oz **baby onions**

4 **garlic cloves**

3 teaspoons **bouillon powder**

about 20 **saffron** threads

salt and pepper

4 tablespoons **olive oil**

2 teaspoons **cinnamon**

2 teaspoons soft **brown sugar**

400 g/14 oz canned **chickpeas**, drained

3 tablespoons **sultanas**

500 g/1 lb 2 oz **couscous**

2 tablespoons chopped fresh **coriander**

NUTRITIONAL INFORMATION one serving contains	
CALORIES:	515
TOTAL FAT:	11.4 G
CARBOHYDRATES:	93.5 G
TOTAL SUGAR:	19.7 G
FIBRE:	8.6 G
SODIUM:	1.1 G

This is a feast of a meal and best eaten in company. Prepare to feel very full indeed,.

METHOD

1. Preheat the oven to 220°C/425°F/gas 7. Prepare all the vegetables: plunge the onions into boiling water for 1 minute, then peel. Put all the vegetables into a very large pan, with the garlic, bouillon, saffron, salt and 2 litres/3½ pints water. Bring to the boil, then simmer for 3–4 minutes. Lift out the vegetables; reserve the stock.

2. Put the carrots, parsnips, pumpkin and onions into a roasting tin and sprinkle on 3 tablespoons olive oil, the cinnamon and sugar, salt and pepper and 5 tablespoons of the vegetable stock.

3. Put the cabbage, leeks and courgettes into another roasting tin and add 1 tablespoon olive oil, 5 tablespoons of the vegetable stock and a little salt and pepper.

4. Put the vegetables into the hot oven, adding the chickpeas and sultanas to the carrots and parsnips after 35 minutes. Continue to roast for a further 10–15 minutes, or until the vegetables are beginning to brown or caramelize.

5. Towards the end of the roasting time, bring the stock back to the boil. Put the couscous in a large bowl and pour over the boiling stock. Leave for about 10 minutes. Loosen with two forks and mix in the coriander. Pile the couscous into a conical shape on a large serving platter.

6. Arrange the vegetables around the couscous.

7. If you have any of the green vegetables left, return them to the stock and serve as an accompaniment. Serve the remaining sweet spiced vegetables in a separate dish.

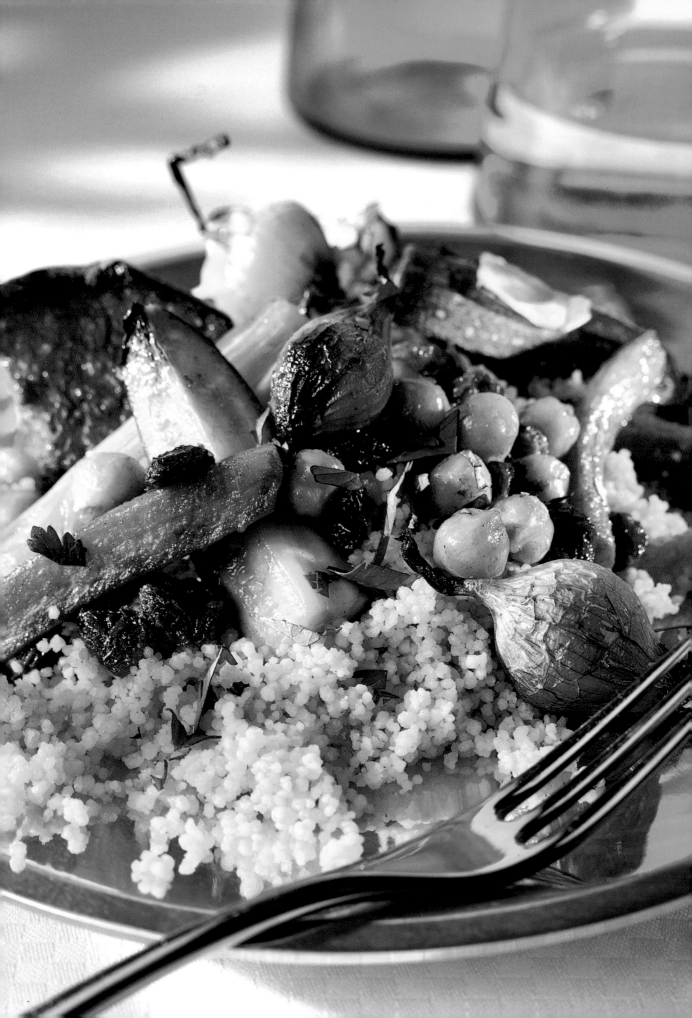

Couscous
with roasted carrots and thyme

SERVES 4

INGREDIENTS

500 g/1 lb 2 oz **carrots**, peeled and cut into
   5 cm/2 inch pieces

¼ small **red onion**, very finely chopped

2 **garlic cloves**, finely sliced

3 sprigs of **thyme**

1 tablespoon **olive oil**

1 teaspoon **tamari**

Basic **couscous** (see page 102 – use
   325 g/12 oz couscous)

I love to make this with organic carrots or young carrots with the green bushy tops that wilt in the heat. If the carrots are small enough you won't need to cut them up. A teaspoon of honey or brown sugar added to the casserole is also in order.

METHOD

1. Preheat the oven to its highest setting.
2. Put the carrots, onion, garlic and thyme into a lidded casserole dish and baste with the oil, tamari and 2 tablespoons hot water. Cover and place in the hot oven for 10–15 minutes.
3. Remove the thyme, turn the carrots over a few times and add a further tablespoon of water. Return to the oven – without the lid – and roast for a further 10–15 minutes, until the carrots are just beginning to caramelize.
4. Towards the end of the roasting time, prepare the couscous.
5. Pile the roasted carrots on top of the couscous and serve hot.

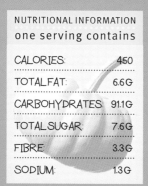

NUTRITIONAL INFORMATION one serving contains	
CALORIES:	450
TOTAL FAT:	6.6 G
CARBOHYDRATES:	91.1 G
TOTAL SUGAR:	7.6 G
FIBRE:	3.3 G
SODIUM:	1.3 G

Spinach, sesame, pineapple
and smoked tofu with couscous

SERVES 4

INGREDIENTS

Basic **couscous** (see page 102 – use
325 g/12 oz couscous)

1 tablespoon **olive oil**

275 g/10 oz **smoked tofu**, cut into julienne
strips

2 tablespoons **tamari**

1 tablespoon **sesame seeds**

1 small can (175 g/6 oz) **pineapple rings** in
natural juice

dash of **Tabasco** sauce

450 g/1 lb baby **spinach**

sea salt

A more Eastern than Middle Eastern combination, that works beautifully. Basmati rice would be a more conventional accompaniment.

METHOD

1. Begin by preparing the couscous: by the time it is soft, the meal will be ready.

2. Heat the oil in a wok or large saucepan, add the tofu strips and stir-fry for 1 minute, turning all the time. Add the tamari and sesame seeds and fry for at least 10 minutes. When the tofu begins to stick, scrape with a metal spoon or spatula to loosen it; the bits that get stuck are the best bits.

3. Add 2 tablespoons of the pineapple juice and fry until the tofu is crisp and dark golden brown. Remove from the pan and keep warm.

4. Add the pineapple rings to the pan, together with the remaining juice, the Tabasco and a dash of tamari. Cook over a high heat until the juice has completely reduced. Remove from the pan and set aside.

5. Add the spinach and a pinch of salt to the pan and stir-fry until the spinach wilts. Remove from the heat, drain off any liquid if necessary and serve at once, topped with the tofu, seeds and pineapple, accompanied by couscous.

NUTRITIONAL INFORMATION
one serving contains

CALORIES:	527
TOTAL FAT:	11.2 G
CARBOHYDRATES:	91.5 G
TOTAL SUGAR:	8.2 G
FIBRE:	2.9 G
SODIUM:	1.8 G

Broccoli, red pepper and asparagus
with hoisin sauce and couscous

SERVES 6

INGREDIENTS

Basic **couscous** (see page 102)

olive oil (see introduction)

500 g/1 lb 2 oz **asparagus spears**

1 **garlic clove**, crushed

500 g/1 lb 2 oz **broccoli**, stalks removed and
    peeled and cut into fine julienne strips

1 **red pepper**, cut into thin strips

1 **yellow pepper**, cut into thin strips

2 tablespoons **hoisin** sauce

½ tablespoon **tamari**

dash of **Tabasco** sauce (optional)

Keep the vegetables crisp and bright. Ideally you would use a spray can of olive oil, which are becoming increasingly available in supermarkets. Otherwise just use a minimum amount of oil: say ½ teaspoon at a time.

METHOD

1. Begin by preparing the couscous: by the time it is soft, the meal will be ready.

2. Heat a wok or large saucepan, add 8 sprays of oil, half the asparagus and half the garlic. Add about 2 tablespoons of water, which will create steam and help to cook the asparagus, and sauté for about 1 minute. Remove the asparagus from the pan; repeat with the rest of the asparagus.

3. Add a further 8 sprays of oil and sauté the broccoli for 1 minute – also in two batches.

4. Remove the broccoli from the pan and add the peppers. Sauté for 30–40 seconds, then remove from the heat.

5. Mix all the vegetables, then return to the wok for a few seconds. Remove from the heat and add the hoisin sauce, tamari and Tabasco to taste. Serve at once, with the couscous.

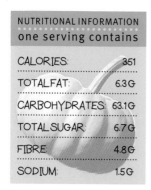

NUTRITIONAL INFORMATION
one serving contains

CALORIES:	351
TOTAL FAT:	6.3 G
CARBOHYDRATES:	63.1 G
TOTAL SUGAR:	6.7 G
FIBRE:	4.8 G
SODIUM:	1.5 G

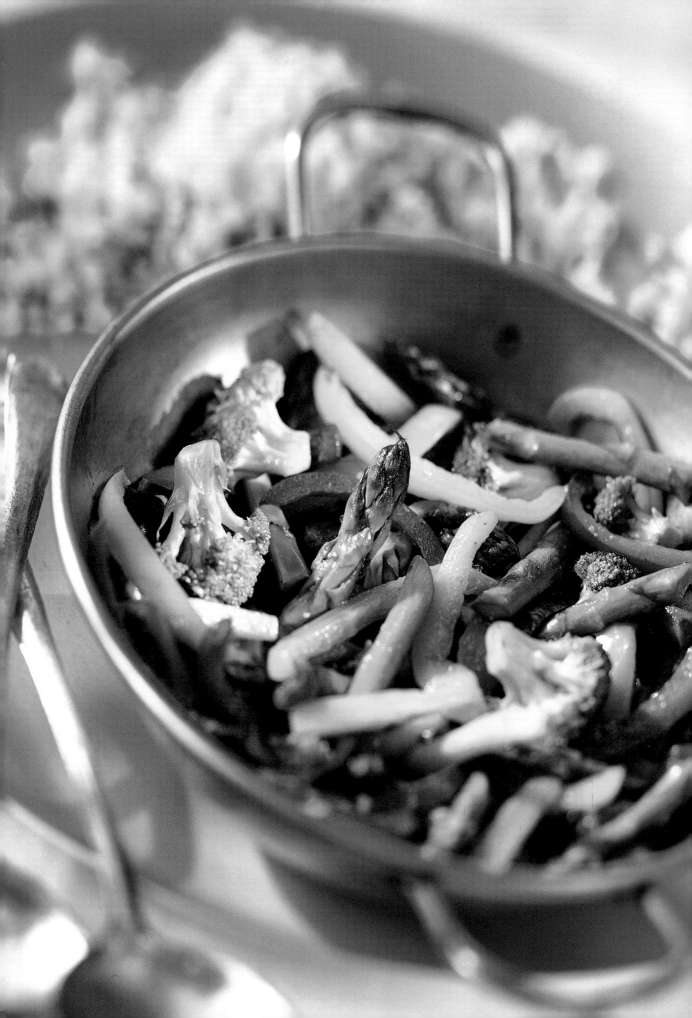

Roasted fennel with couscous

SERVES 4

INGREDIENTS

6 small **fennel** bulbs

2 **garlic cloves**, thinly sliced

1 tablespoon **olive oil**

1 tablespoon **Pernod** (optional)

sea salt and freshly ground black pepper

Basic **couscous** (see page 102 – use 325 g/12 oz couscous)

As anyone familiar with my cooking knows, I love fennel and would not think twice of making a whole meal of it. You could also simply braise the fennel in a heavy-based pan, covered with a little stock and oil, together with finely sliced garlic, and some salt and pepper. Cook over a gentle heat until meltingly tender.

METHOD

1. Preheat the oven to 200°C/400°F/gas 6. Trim the fennel and cut lengthways into four or six pieces, depending on its size.
2. Place the fennel in a roasting tin, interspersing the garlic slices so they are not directly exposed to the heat. Baste with the oil and Pernod, if using. Sprinkle with salt and pepper and place in the hot oven for 20–25 minutes, until tender and beginning to char.
3. Towards the end of the roasting time, prepare the couscous. Pile the roasted fennel on top of the couscous and serve hot.

NUTRITIONAL INFORMATION
one serving contains

CALORIES:	455
TOTAL FAT:	6.7 G
CARBOHYDRATES:	89.2 G
TOTAL SUGAR:	6.6 G
FIBRE:	9.1 G
SODIUM:	1.5 G

Spiced pumpkin and chickpea couscous

SERVES 6–8

INGREDIENTS

1 **pumpkin** (about 3–4 kg/8 lb), seeds removed,
   cut into 5 cm x 2 cm/2 inch x ¾ inch chunks

1 teaspoon ground **ginger**

a good pinch of **nutmeg**

1½ teaspoons ground **cinnamon**

2 teaspoons soft **brown sugar**

a good pinch of salt

2 tablespoons **olive oil**

a dash of **Tabasco** sauce

400 g/14 oz canned **chickpeas**, drained

100 g/3½ oz **raisins**, soaked in boiling water for
   a few minutes, then drained

Basic **couscous** (see page 102)

2 tablespoons chopped fresh **parsley**

Traditionally, this is served after a meat-based couscous, together with other sweet vegetables, but when you try it you will see that it is a sumptuous meal in itself.

METHOD

1. Preheat the oven to 200°C/400°F/gas 6. Put the pumpkin in a roasting tin. Mix together the spices, sugar, salt, oil and Tabasco and use about half of this mixture to baste the pumpkin. Cover with foil and roast for 20–25 minutes.

2. Remove the foil and add the chickpeas and raisins, together with the remaining spice mixture. Turn the pumpkin to coat it with the spice mixture, then return to the oven for a further 20–25 minutes, until caramelized.

3. Towards the end of the roasting time, prepare the couscous. Pile the spiced roasted vegetables on top of the couscous, sprinkle with parsley and serve hot.

NUTRITIONAL INFORMATION
one serving contains

CALORIES:	486
TOTAL FAT:	8 G
CARBOHYDRATES:	93.8 G
TOTAL SUGAR:	18.9 G
FIBRE:	7.5 G
SODIUM:	1.1 G

Christmas vegetables with cranberries
on a bed of couscous

SERVES 8

INGREDIENTS

275 g/10 oz **tofu**, cut into 3 cm/1 inch cubes

100 g/3½ oz **dried cranberries**

500 g/1 lb 2 oz **parsnips**

500 g/1 lb 2 oz **carrots**

500 g/1 lb 2 oz **sweet potatoes**

500 g/1 lb 2 oz new **potatoes**

500 g/1 lb 2 oz **baby onions**

1 tablespoon **olive oil**

Basic **couscous** (see page 102)

TOFU MARINADE

6 tablespoons **tamari**

1 tablespoon **brandy**

1 tablespoon **olive oil**

½ teaspoon **Tabasco sauce**

VEGETABLE MARINADE

1 tablespoon **tamari**

juice of ½ **orange**

1 tablespoon chopped **fresh coriander**

1 tablespoon **brandy**

1 **garlic clove**, crushed

NUTRITIONAL INFORMATION one serving contains	
CALORIES:	566
TOTAL FAT:	10.3 G
CARBOHYDRATES:	106.4 G
TOTAL SUGAR:	15.9 G
FIBRE:	7.9 G
SODIUM:	3 G

Serve any leftover tofu marinade hot and use to douse the couscous.

METHOD

1. Mix the ingredients for the tofu marinade with 6 tablespoons water. Add the tofu and leave for 1 hour.
2. Mix the ingredients for the vegetable marinade with 100 ml/3½ fl oz water and salt and pepper to taste, add the cranberries and leave to soak.
3. Preheat the oven to 220°C/425°F/gas 7.
4. Peel the parsnips, carrots and sweet potatoes and cut into 1 cm/½ inch thick diagonal slices. Halve or quarter the new potatoes. Blanch the parsnips and carrots in boiling water for about 45 seconds. Drain, refresh and drain well.
5. Strain the cranberries and set aside. Put the parsnips, carrots and baby onions into a casserole dish, pour over half the vegetable marinade, cover with a tightly fitting lid and bake for about 40 minutes.
6. Put the potatoes and sweet potatoes on a roasting tray with 1 tablespoon olive oil and the remaining marinade; roast for 20 minutes.
7. Drain the tofu, reserving the marinade, and roast in the oven for 20 minutes, basting and turning every 5 minutes.
8. Transfer the parsnips, carrots and onions to the roasting tray with the potatoes and roast all together for a further 20 minutes.
9. Towards the end of the roasting time, prepare the couscous.
10. Add the cranberries to the vegetables for the last 5–6 minutes of the roasting time.
11. Pile the tofu on top of a bed of roasted vegetables and serve hot, with couscous.

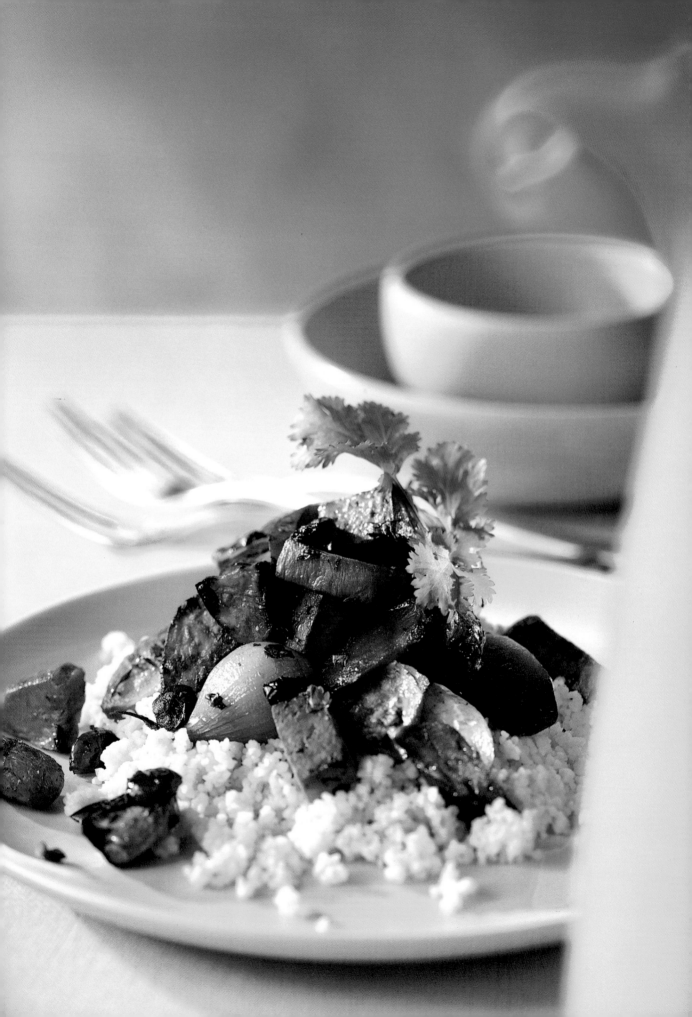

DRINKS

For truly instant **vitality**, what could be more natural than grabbing a drink? But let's get one thing clear – we are not talking about a cup of tea or even a designer coffee; they may seem to **boost** your energy for a short time, but in the long term they'll fill your body with toxins that it doesn't need. Fruit and vegetables are bursting with vitamins and minerals, contain practically zero fat, and can be **blended** with each other or with yoghurt or sparkling mineral water to create totally cool, terrifically **energizing** drinks.

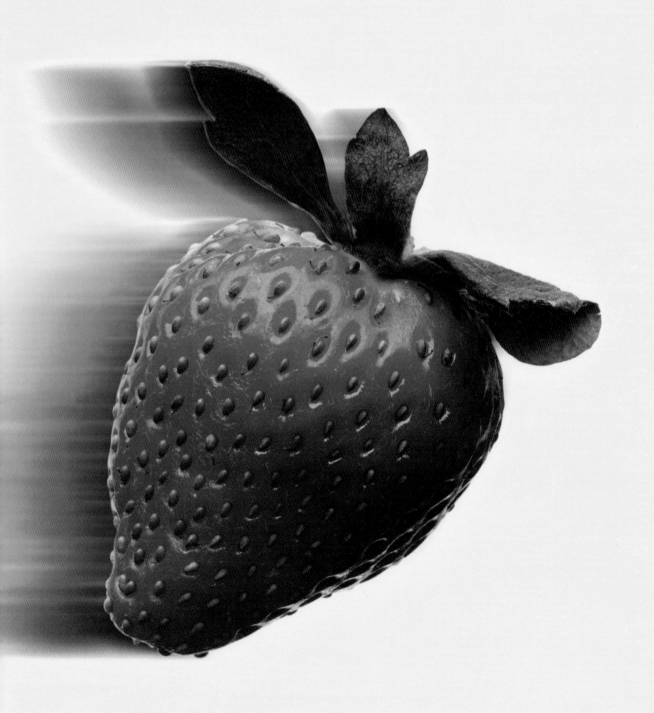

Tropical fruit lassi

SERVES 4

INGREDIENTS

about 10 **ice cubes**

500 g/1 lb 2 oz low-fat **bio yoghurt**

1 ripe **papaya**, peeled and seeded

1 large ripe **mango**, peeled and seeded

1 **passion fruit**

Lassi is a traditional Indian yoghurt drink. Sold in roadside stalls as well as fabulous juice bars, lassis offer cool relief to the hot weather and are perfect served with spicy food. Salt lassis, which at first seem odd to the Western palate, are in fact fantastically refreshing. Anyone who has tried in vain to cool their mouth with water after a particularly spicy meal will appreciate the way in which yoghurt drinks do the trick. I am told that this is because capsiacin, the chemical that makes chillies hot, is not water soluble, whereas it is effectively dissolved by milky or yoghurty drinks.

METHOD

1. Crush the ice and place in a blender. Add the yoghurt, papaya and mango. Cut the passion fruit in half and scrape the juice and pulp into the blender. Blend until smooth, pour into a jug and serve at once.

NUTRITIONAL INFORMATION one serving contains	
CALORIES:	227
TOTAL FAT:	2.2 G
CARBOHYDRATES:	42.1 G
TOTAL SUGAR:	42 G
FIBRE:	6.8 G
SODIUM:	0.4 G

Coconut and lime lassi

SERVES 4

INGREDIENTS

about 18 **ice cubes**

600 g/1¼ lb low-fat **yoghurt**

400 ml/14 fl oz unsweetened **coconut milk**

1 **lime**

2–3 tablespoons **icing sugar**

Coconut and lime are natural companions. The crushed ice is crucial, but you can play with the proportions to suit yourself.

METHOD

1. Crush the ice and place in a large jug.
2. Put the yoghurt and coconut milk into a blender. Use a lemon zester to pare off the lime zest. Squeeze the juice from the lime, scrape out the pulp and add both to the blender. Blend for 1 minute, add icing sugar to taste and blend briefly. Pour into the jug and serve at once, garnished with the lime zest.

NUTRITIONAL INFORMATION
one serving contains

CALORIES:	144
TOTAL FAT:	1.5 G
CARBOHYDRATES:	26.2 G
TOTAL SUGAR:	26 G
FIBRE:	0
SODIUM:	0.6 G

Rosewater and cardamom lassi
with pomegranate

SERVES 4–6

INGREDIENTS

4 **pomegranates**

800 g/1¾ lb low-fat **yoghurt**

1 teaspoon **rosewater essence**

1 **cardamom pod**, seeds removed and finely
  ground in a pestle and mortar

4 tablespoons water

2–3 teaspoons **icing sugar**

Rosewater is a typically Indian flavour, which I find marries particularly well with pomegranate, while providing a perfect home for a difficult-to-eat fruit. Like most lassis and yoghurt drinks this must be served very cold. I have sometimes added crushed ice to it, but this tends to dilute the delicate flavours; I'd rather just make sure that the yoghurt was well chilled. The flavour of rosewater is brought out by sugar, but taste the lassi before sweetening. Also go easy on the cardamom: a very few seeds suffice. The yoghurt should be smooth, not the set variety.

METHOD

1. Squeeze the juice of three of the pomegranates through a strainer into a large jug. Scoop the seeds of the remaining pomegranate and add to the jug.
2. Add all the other ingredients, with icing sugar to taste, stir well and serve at once.

NUTRITIONAL INFORMATION
one serving contains

CALORIES	151
TOTAL FAT	1.3 G
CARBOHYDRATES	28.1 G
TOTAL SUGAR	28 G
FIBRE	4.5 G
SODIUM	0.3 G

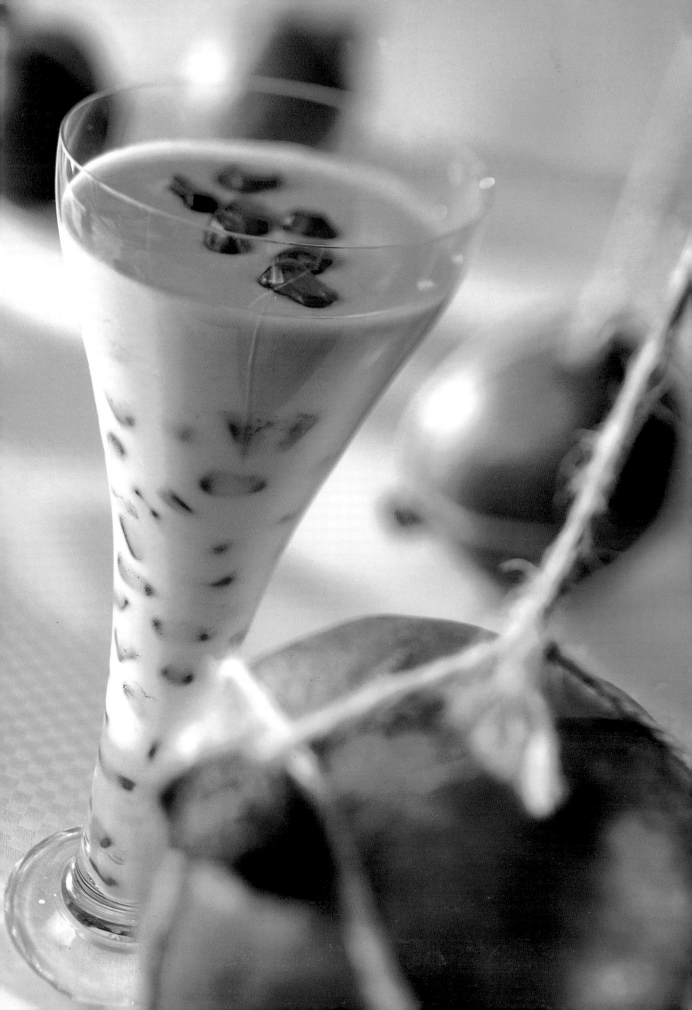

Apple, carrot and beetroot frappé

SERVES 6

INGREDIENTS

6 large **carrots**, peeled and trimmed

1 large **beetroot**, peeled and trimmed

2 **apples**, cut into quarters

about 18 **ice cubes**

dash of **Tabasco** sauce (optional)

pinch of freshly grated **nutmeg**

sea salt and freshly ground black pepper

You will need a juicer to make this super-healthy drink. It provides a powerful hit of vitamins; so much so that you may want to dilute it slightly with mineral water. Vitamins oxygenate the body, so you will feel almost as if you have been for a run in the woods after drinking it. Come to think of it, it is brilliant after a run in the woods.

METHOD

1. Put the carrots, beetroot and apples through a juicer.
2. Crush the ice and place in a blender, then add the vegetable juice and blend for a few seconds. Season to taste with Tabasco, nutmeg, salt and pepper and serve immediately.

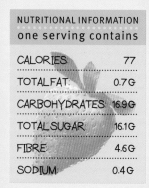

NUTRITIONAL INFORMATION
one serving contains

CALORIES:	77
TOTAL FAT:	0.7 G
CARBOHYDRATES:	16.9 G
TOTAL SUGAR:	16.1 G
FIBRE:	4.6 G
SODIUM:	0.4 G

Melon, kiwi and strawberry drink

SERVES 4

INGREDIENTS

1 large **melon** (e.g. honeydew)

3 **kiwi fruit**

125 g/4 oz **strawberries**

Light, refreshing, a magical combination of flavours. Both kiwi fruit and strawberries are full of vitamin C, so this is a great vitality booster.

METHOD

1. Cut the melon in half, discard the seeds, then scoop the flesh into a blender.
2. Peel the kiwi fruit and add to the blender, together with the strawberries. Blend and chill.

NUTRITIONAL INFORMATION
one serving contains

CALORIES	57
TOTAL FAT	0.4 G
CARBOHYDRATES	12.9 G
TOTAL SUGAR	12.8 G
FIBRE	1.8 G
SODIUM	0.1 G

Peach and strawberry smoothie

SERVES 4–6

INGREDIENTS

8 ripe **peaches**, stones removed

1 punnet (250 g/9 oz) **strawberries**

1 **guava** (optional)

caster sugar (optional)

This is a dairy-free smoothie with body and texture. Ripe fruit is always preferable, but you will be amazed at how juicing can extract flavour you wouldn't have known was there. A juicer is brilliant for this, so that you really get a drink and not just a fruit pulp. I had to test this recipe in the winter with out-of-season strawberries and still the fragrance of strawberries filled the house all morning. Try adding a guava for an even more special perfume.

METHOD

1. Put all the fruit through a juicer. Taste and add a little sugar if necessary – I didn't need it. Mix well and refrigerate until ready to serve.

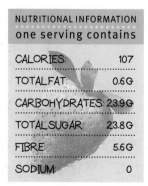

NUTRITIONAL INFORMATION
one serving contains

CALORIES:	107
TOTAL FAT:	0.6G
CARBOHYDRATES:	23.9G
TOTAL SUGAR:	23.8G
FIBRE:	5.6G
SODIUM:	0

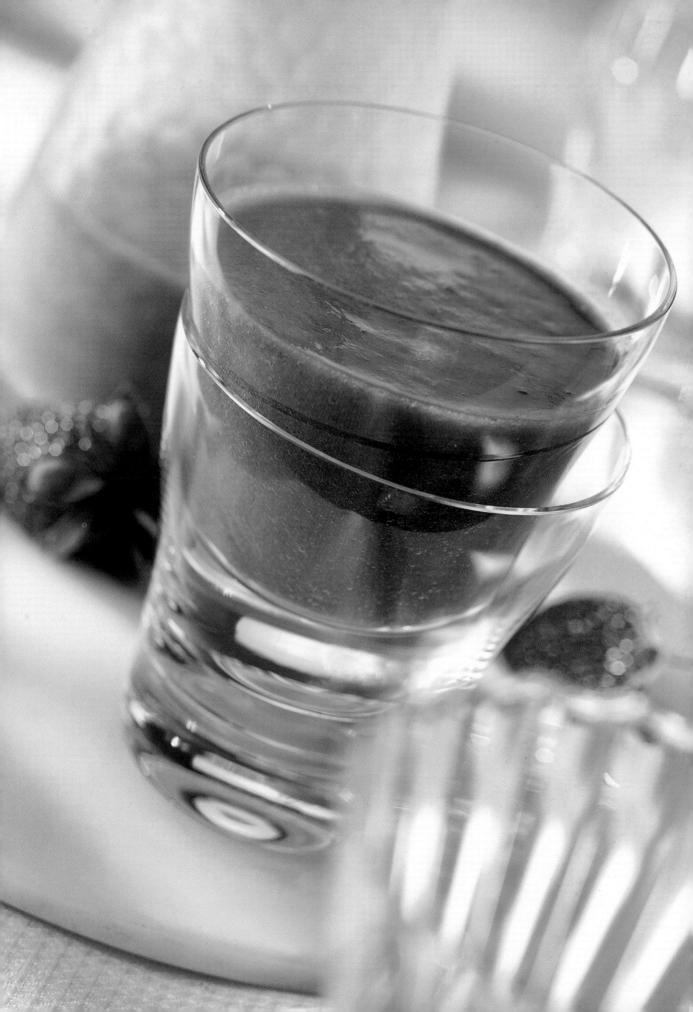

Blackberry smoothie

SERVES 4

INGREDIENTS

250 g/9 oz frozen **blackberries**

500 g/1 lb 2 oz low-fat **yoghurt**

2 tablespoons **caster sugar**

You can make this with frozen blackberries or frozen raspberries, but then you will probably need to increase the sugar content. It is a wonderful way to use fresh blackberries that you have picked from a hedge in autumn. Leave a few blackberries whole to sink to the bottom as a last-moment treat.

METHOD

1. Put all the ingredients in a blender and blend briefly, creating a marbled effect. Serve at once.

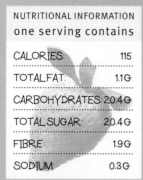

NUTRITIONAL INFORMATION one serving contains	
CALORIES	115
TOTAL FAT	1.1 G
CARBOHYDRATES	20.4 G
TOTAL SUGAR	20.4 G
FIBRE	1.9 G
SODIUM	0.3 G

Banana yoghurt breakfast smoothie

INGREDIENTS

500 g/1 lb 2 oz low-fat **bio yoghurt**

85 g/3 oz **muesli**

2 **bananas**, peeled

1 tablespoon **honey**

No time to sit down to breakfast? Start your day with a smoothie instead. This tastes best if it is not too cold.

METHOD

1. Put all the ingredients in a blender with 2 tablespoons of water and blend until smooth.

NUTRITIONAL INFORMATION
one serving contains

CALORIES:	207
TOTAL FAT:	2.5 G
CARBOHYDRATES:	39.4 G
TOTAL SUGAR:	27.4 G
FIBRE:	0.5 G
SODIUM:	0.3 G

DESSERTS

It is much easier than you might think to make **low-fat** desserts without being restricted to the fruit bowl. Even a dessert traditionally oozing with butter such as an apple charlotte can be absolutely **delicious** with much less – and chocolate need not be entirely banished to some culinary gulag. What has all but disappeared is the cream and the butter, yet yoghurt or buttermilk create a creaminess which is, if anything, more delicious as well as being so much **easier** for the body to handle. Maple syrup is a rich, natural alternative to sugar with nothing like its addictive properties, and the potential of **exotic** fruit for adding its own fresh sweetness is also explored.

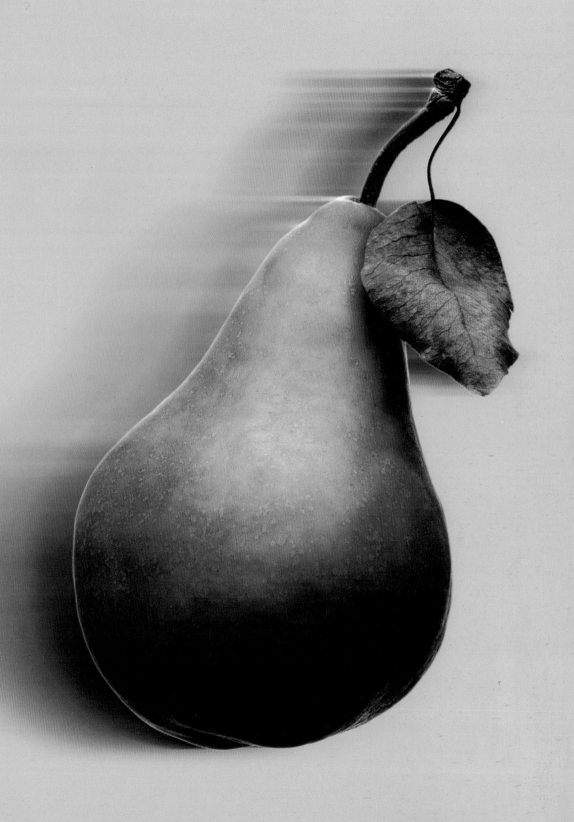

Dates
with whipped ricotta and orange sauce

SERVES 4

INGREDIENTS
12–16 fresh **dates** (preferably Medjool)

85 g/3 oz **ricotta**

85 g/3 oz **fromage frais**

2 teaspoons **elderflower cordial**, or

   2 teaspoons caster sugar

ORANGE SAUCE
100 ml/3½ fl oz fresh **orange juice**

1 tablespoon **brandy**

2 tablespoons **sugar**

Dates have a particular sweetness which matches the intensity of chocolate and can make a pretty good substitute for it when the occasion demands. This simple, satisfying dessert can be made with ricotta or fromage frais alone, although I like the half-and-half mixture. Elderflower cordial adds a delicate sweetness, but sugar can be used instead.

METHOD
1. Split the dates and remove the stones.
2. Beat the ricotta, fromage frais and cordial or sugar together until light and fluffy and use to fill the dates.
3. Simmer the orange juice with the brandy and sugar for a couple of minutes.
4. Arrange the filled dates on individual serving plates and spoon the orange sauce over them.

NUTRITIONAL INFORMATION
one serving contains

CALORIES:	232
TOTAL FAT:	3.9G
CARBOHYDRATES:	44.9G
TOTAL SUGAR:	44.9G
FIBRE:	1.8G
SODIUM:	0.1G

Grilled pineapple
with fragrant coconut milk

SERVES 4

INGREDIENTS
1 large ripe **pineapple**

4 tablespoons **soft brown sugar**

FRAGRANT COCONUT MILK
200 ml/7 fl oz **coconut milk**

2 teaspoons **caster sugar**

juice of ¼ **lime**

zest of ½ **lime**

seeds from 1 **cardamom pod**

2 cm/¾ inch **lemongrass**, cut lengthways into
   thin strips

Serve this hot, each individual pineapple boat sitting in a pool of sauce. Use a cannelling knife to make thin strips of lime zest – and do use a ripe pineapple.

METHOD
1. Put all the ingredients for the fragrant coconut milk into a saucepan and simmer for 5 minutes. Remove from the heat and leave to infuse for 30 minutes.

2. Preheat the oven to 200°C/400°F/gas 6. Preheat the grill to medium. Cut the pineapple into quarters lengthways, leaving on the skin and leafy top. Remove the core. Run a knife between the flesh and the skin to free the flesh, then slice the flesh into sections, still keeping it in the skin. Sprinkle with the sugar and place under the grill until golden brown in places.

3. Place the grilled pineapple boats in an ovenproof dish. Strain the coconut milk if you like, then pour it around the pineapple boats and place in the hot oven until the coconut milk is bubbling. Serve hot.

NUTRITIONAL INFORMATION one serving contains	
CALORIES:	127
TOTAL FAT:	0.4G
CARBOHYDRATES:	32.9G
TOTAL SUGAR:	32.9G
FIBRE:	1.5G
SODIUM:	0.2G

Apple and mango filo tart

SERVES 6

INGREDIENTS

1 kg/2¼ lb dessert **apples**, peeled, cored and
thinly sliced

100 ml/3½ fl oz **apple juice**

1 large or 2 small ripe **mangoes**

300 g/11 oz **filo pastry**

2 teaspoons **sunflower** or **rapeseed oil**

½–1 teaspoon **icing sugar**

With fragrant apples and a ripe mango the flavours merge gently together, and I needed to use very little sugar in this recipe, but follow your own taste buds. Sunflower oil is sometimes sold in a spray can; this makes it easier to oil the filo pastry sparingly.

METHOD

1. Heat the oven to 200°C/400°F/gas 6.
2. Simmer the apples in the apple juice until just tender; the liquid should be reduced and slightly thickened. Meanwhile, peel the mango and slice thinly.
3. Arrange four sheets of filo pastry in a 25 cm/ 10 inch diameter loose-bottomed tart tin, brushing or spraying each sheet lightly with oil. Place in the oven for 5–10 minutes, until the pastry is crisp and pale golden. The tart can be prepared ahead up to this point.
4. Fill the tart with the prepared fruit. Divide the remaining filo pastry sheets into quarters, scrunch up loosely and arrange over the fruit. Spray or drizzle a little more oil over the top and bake for 20–25 minutes, until golden brown.
5. Leave to cool for about 5 minutes, then dust lightly with icing sugar and serve warm.

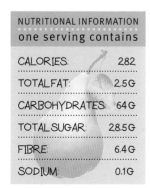

NUTRITIONAL INFORMATION
one serving contains

CALORIES:	282
TOTAL FAT:	2.5G
CARBOHYDRATES:	64G
TOTAL SUGAR:	28.5G
FIBRE:	6.4G
SODIUM:	0.1G

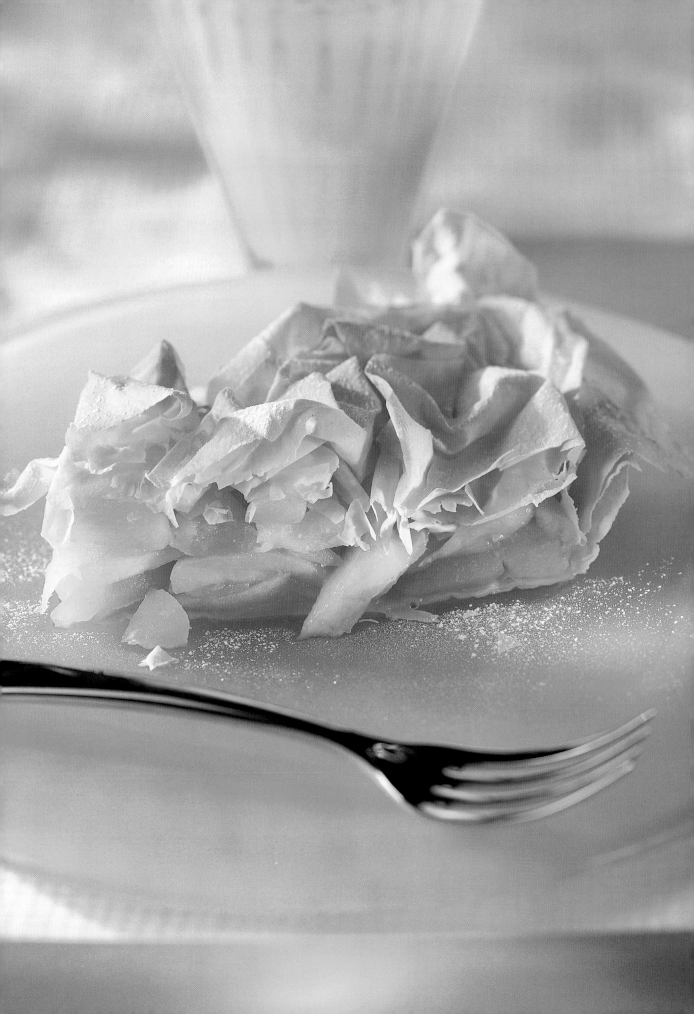

Fruit salad with mango sauce

SERVES 4–6

INGREDIENTS

3 **nectarines**, halved, stones removed

1 small **cantaloupe melon**, halved, seeds
removed

1 **papaya**, peeled, halved, seeds removed

2 **passion fruit**, halved, juice sieved

½ punnet of **blueberries** (85 g/3 oz)

MANGO SAUCE

1 very large (650 g/1 lb 6 oz) **mango** or 2 small
mangoes

I have made this with exotic fruit, but fragrant
apples, ripe sweet pears and other seasonal fruit
could be used to great effect in this way, livened up
by a fruit sauce. Instead of the mango the sauce
could be made of puréed berries. It's a great way to
start the day and to speed up your metabolism.

METHOD

1. To make the mango sauce, peel the mangoes and
   scrape the flesh off the stones, holding them over
   the blender as you do so to catch all the juice.
   Blend the flesh with 100 ml/3½ fl oz water until
   smooth, then chill.
2. Cut the nectarines, melon and papaya into thin
   slices and arrange on individual plates. Pour
   over the passion fruit juice and scatter over the
   blueberries. Pour the chilled mango sauce
   around the plate.

NUTRITIONAL INFORMATION
one serving contains

CALORIES:	160
TOTAL FAT:	0.7 G
CARBOHYDRATES:	37.2 G
TOTAL SUGAR:	30.2 G
FIBRE:	8.6 G
SODIUM:	0.1 G

Tropical fruit kebabs

SERVES 4

INGREDIENTS

1 tablespoon **maple syrup**

½ tablespoon **brandy**

1 small **pineapple**

1 **papaya**, ripe but firm

1 **mango**, ripe but firm

4 small **bananas**

1 **star fruit**

mint leaves, to decorate

MAPLE YOGHURT SAUCE

4 tablespoons **maple syrup**

3 teaspoons **brandy**

150 g/5 oz low-fat **bio yoghurt**

This must be made with good-quality ripe fruit and can look exotic and exquisite. A cheap blowtorch from a hardware store is a great investment: it means you can caramelize sugars and brown the tops of puddings very quickly, giving a charred look that isn't always possible just through grilling. However, you can cook this on a barbecue or under a grill, but whichever way you choose, be sure to cook the kebabs on a sheet of thick foil in order to catch the delicious juices.

METHOD

1. Place four long wooden skewers in a dish of water and leave to soak for at least 1 hour.

2. Preheat the grill. Mix the maple syrup and brandy together. Cut the pineapple into thick slices, then into wedges, leaving the skin on. Cut the papaya in half and scoop out the seeds, then cut into quarters, leaving the skin on. Cut the large flat stone out of the mango, then cut the mango into quarters, leaving the skin on. Peel the bananas, then pull the skins back over the fruit. Cut the star fruit into four thick slices.

3. Arrange the fruit on the skewers and place on the grill rack. Brush with the maple syrup mixture and grill for 15 minutes, turning occasionally, until starting to brown.

4. Mix the sauce ingredients together to a thin pouring consistency, adding the juices from the kebabs. Serve one kebab per person, with a little of the sauce drizzled over. Garnish with mint leaves and serve the remaining sauce separately.

NUTRITIONAL INFORMATION one serving contains	
CALORIES:	320
TOTAL FAT:	1.1 G
CARBOHYDRATES:	73.9 G
TOTAL SUGAR:	65.4 G
FIBRE:	7.1 G
SODIUM:	0.2 G

Poached pears with chocolate sauce

SERVES 6

INGREDIENTS

6 firm dessert **pears**

300 ml/10 fl oz **rosé wine**

150 ml/5 fl oz **apple juice**

4 **cloves**

1 **cinnamon stick**

1 **bay leaf**

4–5 tablespoons **caster sugar**

CHOCOLATE SAUCE

125 g/4 oz good-quality **dark chocolate**
  (70% cocoa solids), chopped

250 ml/8 fl oz boiling water

85 g/3 oz **cocoa powder**

85 g/3 oz **caster sugar**

This is a classic combination. The fibre of the pear helps the chocolate go down, guilt-free. And the chocolate sauce is dairy-free, which makes it easier on the fat front.

METHOD

1. Peel, halve and core the pears.
2. Put the wine and apple juice into a saucepan just large enough to hold the pears in a single layer. Add the cloves, cinnamon, bay leaf and sugar and bring to the boil.
3. Add the pears, reduce the heat, cover with a lid and simmer for 6–7 minutes, or until the pears are tender when tested with a metal skewer. Lift the pears out of the liquid with a slotted spoon and leave to drain.
4. For the sauce, put the chocolate and 175 ml/ 6 fl oz boiling water into a bowl set over a saucepan of hot water and stir until smooth. Dissolve the cocoa powder and sugar in 75 ml/ 3 fl oz boiling water to form a thick paste. Mix with the melted chocolate mixture and pour over the pears. Serve warm.

NUTRITIONAL INFORMATION one serving contains	
CALORIES:	345
TOTAL FAT:	9G
CARBOHYDRATES:	58.1G
TOTAL SUGAR:	56.2G
FIBRE:	5.2G
SODIUM:	0.4G

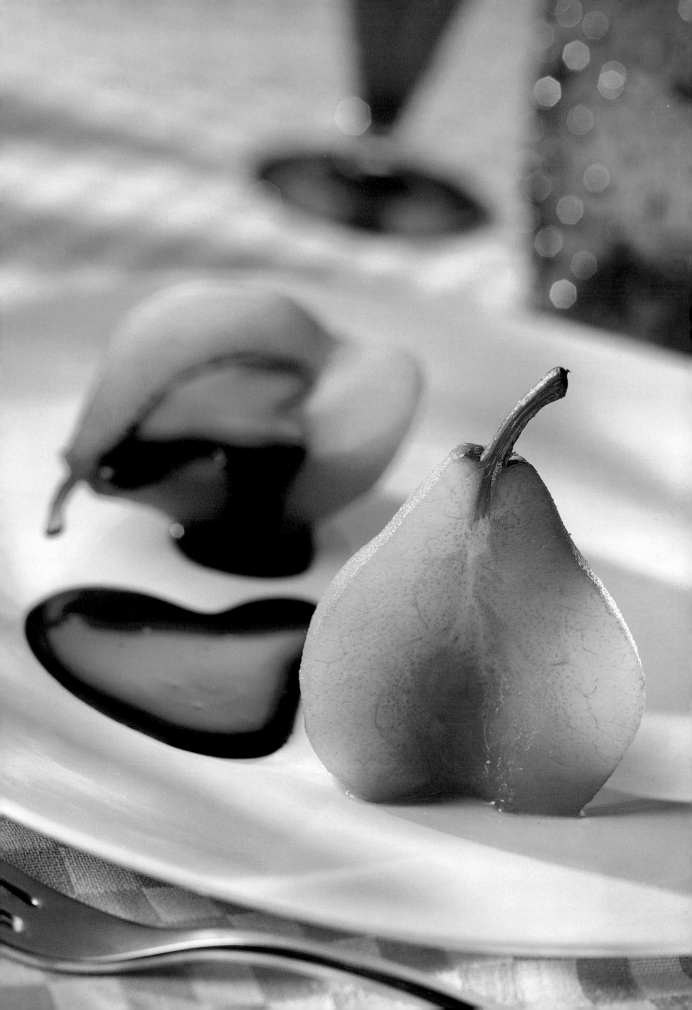

Pear and fig charlotte

SERVES 6

INGREDIENTS
3 **dried figs**, cut into thin slices

325 ml/12 fl oz unsweetened **apple juice**

150 ml/5 fl oz **brandy**

900 g/2 lb **ripe pears**, peeled, cored and sliced

2 tablespoons **maple syrup**

200 g/7 oz sliced **white bread**, crusts removed

25 g/1 oz **butter**

This uses less than a quarter of the butter usually associated with a charlotte, and meets our low fat criteria, managing to come out pleasantly rich and sweet – and much lighter and easier on the stomach. Serve hot or cold.

METHOD
1. Heat the oven to 200°C/400°F/gas 6.
2. Put the figs in a saucepan with 250 ml/8 fl oz of the apple juice and 125 ml/4 fl oz of the brandy and simmer for about 5 minutes, then add the pears, cover and simmer for about 15 minutes, until the pears are tender. Stir in 1 tablespoon of the maple syrup.
3. Trim the bread to fit the base and sides of a 1.5 litre/2½ pint soufflé dish. Put the remaining apple juice, brandy and the butter in a small saucepan and bring to the boil, to emulsify the butter. Brush the liquid lightly over the bread and use to line the soufflé dish, butter side out.
4. Using a slotted spoon, put the pear mixture into the dish, cover with more bread and spoon the liquid over the top, together with the remaining maple syrup. Bake until the top is crisp, about 40–45 minutes. Serve warm.

NUTRITIONAL INFORMATION
one serving contains

CALORIES:	281
TOTAL FAT:	4.4 G
CARBOHYDRATES:	45.4 G
TOTAL SUGAR:	29.5 G
FIBRE:	4.5 G
SODIUM:	0.6 G

Autumn pudding

SERVES 6

INGREDIENTS

150 g/5 oz **blackberries**

2 tablespoons **caster sugar**

225 g/8 oz ripe **plums**, stoned and sliced

225 g/8 oz ripe **pears**, peeled, cored and sliced

225 g/8 oz dessert **apples**, peeled, cored and
  sliced

200 ml/7 fl oz unsweetened **apple juice**

pinch of ground **cinnamon**

300 g/11 oz **sliced white bread**, crusts
  removed

100 ml ml/3½ fl oz **red grape juice** (or apple
  juice blended with a few blackberries)

Like a good summer pudding this must be moist and positively stuffed with fruit. Fortunately, berries freeze very well, a bonus in all seasons, so you can make this even in winter – and it's virtually fat free. I made it as low in sugar as possible, but you should taste the fruits as you prepare them and add more sugar if they seem tart.

METHOD

1. Sprinkle the blackberries with 2 teaspoons sugar and set aside.
2. Stew the plums with 1 heaped tablespoon sugar and 2 tablespoons water, until tender.
3. In separate saucepans, simmer the pears and apples in 100 ml/3½ fl oz apple juice. Taste the apples and add cinnamon and 1 teaspoon sugar, or sweeten to taste.
4. Trim the bread and line the base and sides of a 1.5 litre/2½ pint soufflé dish. Moisten the bread with red grape juice.
5. Add the pears, then a layer of bread, the blackberries, a layer of bread, the apples, and a layer of bread, moistening each layer with juice. Add the plums, cover with bread and spoon over the remaining juice. Cover with a plate and a weight and leave overnight in the refrigerator.
6. To serve, turn out and slice.

NUTRITIONAL INFORMATION
one serving contains

CALORIES:	211
TOTAL FAT:	1.2 G
CARBOHYDRATES:	48.3 G
TOTAL SUGAR:	25 G
FIBRE:	3.6 G
SODIUM:	0.7 G

Roasted apple bananas
with kumquat confit

SERVES 4

INGREDIENTS

500 g/1 lb 2 oz **kumquats**

1 kg/2¼ lb apple **bananas**

5 tablespoons **soft brown sugar**

1 tablespoon **maple syrup** (or extra sugar)

2 tablespoons **brandy**

2 tablespoons water

YOGHURT SAUCE

6 tablespoons **yoghurt**, sieved

1 tablespoon **maple syrup**

Apple bananas are those tiny bananas you often see in Asian supermarkets and increasingly in mainstream ones. You can use ordinary bananas for this dessert – it works just as well. Kumquats, which look like tiny oranges, have a topsy turvy taste – it is their skins which are sweet and their centres sour. They are fantastic caramelized and hold their jewel shape. Here is another dessert that is low in fat and rich in vitamin C.

METHOD

1. Preheat the oven to 200°C/400°F/gas 6.
2. Cut the kumquats in half and remove the seeds. Put the sugar, brandy and water in a saucepan over a low heat, until the sugar dissolves. Add the kumquats and simmer for about 10 minutes.
3. Meanwhile, roast the bananas for 15–20 minutes, until the skins are quite black and the bananas are very soft.
4. Mix the yoghurt and maple syrup for the sauce.
5. Peel the bananas and arrange on four large serving plates. Spoon the kumquats and their syrup around the bananas. To serve, gently pour some of the yoghurt sauce on either side of the kumquats.

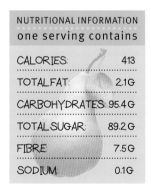

NUTRITIONAL INFORMATION
one serving contains

CALORIES:	413
TOTAL FAT:	2.1G
CARBOHYDRATES:	95.4G
TOTAL SUGAR:	89.2G
FIBRE:	7.5G
SODIUM:	0.1G

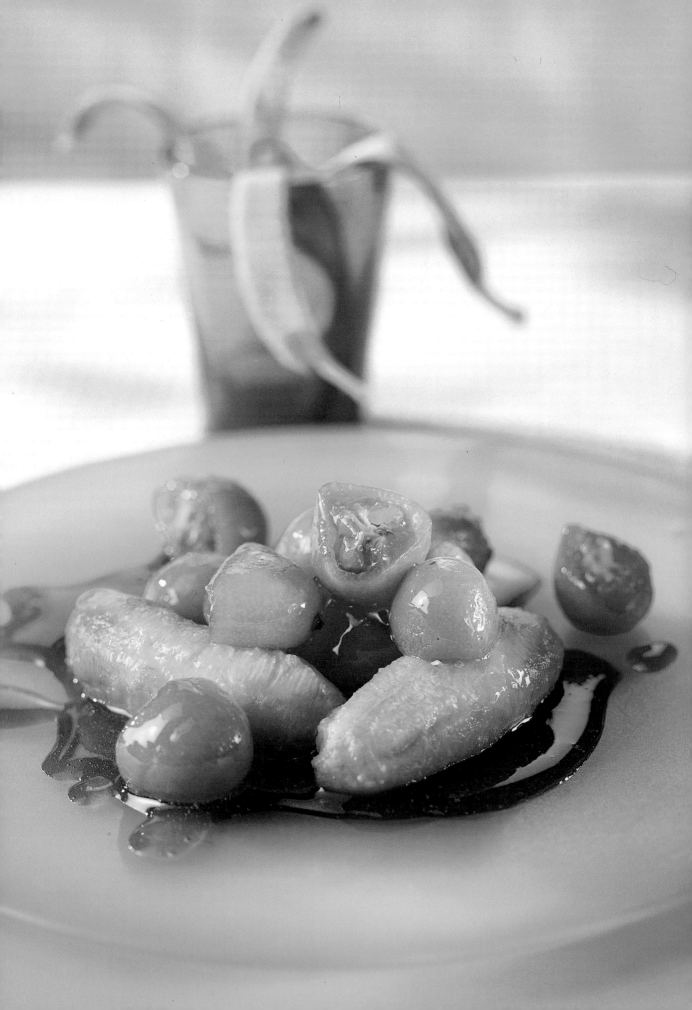

Iced strawberry, meringue
and yoghurt fool

SERVES 4

INGREDIENTS
3 **egg whites**
pinch of **cornflour**
175 g/6 oz **caster sugar**
250 g/9 oz **strawberries**
250 g/9 oz low-fat **bio yoghurt**

Crush the strawberries quite lightly and eat this just partly frozen – the flavours will merge and the dessert will seem remarkably rich, although in fact it's very low in fat and the strawberries provide masses of vitamin C.

You will need only six meringues for this recipe; the rest can be frozen and served with other fruit desserts.

METHOD

1. Heat the oven to 100°C/200°F/gas ¼ or its lowest setting. Line a baking sheet with baking parchment and grease it very lightly with sunflower oil.
2. Put the egg whites in a bowl and beat with the mixer at its highest setting, adding the cornflour after a few seconds. Whisk until the whites hold firm peaks, then add the sugar a tablespoon at a time, whisking all the time.
3. Use a dessertspoon to shape 12–14 meringues, gently spooning them on to the baking paper. Bake until crisp, about 1 hour. Turn off the oven and open the door, leaving the meringues to cool in the oven.
4. Blend the strawberries to a coarse purée. Tip into a bowl and add the yoghurt. Crumble in six of the meringues and mix together. Pour into a freezerproof bowl and freeze until almost solid, about 45 minutes, stirring once or twice.
5. To serve, stir to mix the frozen parts with the liquid, then divide between four stemmed glasses and serve at once.

NUTRITIONAL INFORMATION one serving contains	
CALORIES:	131
TOTAL FAT:	0.7 G
CARBOHYDRATES:	28.2 G
TOTAL SUGAR:	28.1 G
FIBRE:	0.7 G
SODIUM:	0.2 G

Coconut rice pudding

SERVES 4-6

INGREDIENTS
1.2 litres/2 pints **milk**
150 g/5 oz **pudding rice**
50 g/2 oz **caster sugar**
pinch of **ground nutmeg**
40 g/1½ oz **creamed coconut**

This has about one-third of the calories of 'normal' rice pudding and is considerably lower in fat, but the coconut and the natural creaminess of the rice make this as rich as it needs to be. It is very good eaten cold topped with finely chopped fruit – fresh or soaked dried.

METHOD
1. Heat the milk to just below boiling point. Add the rice, sugar, nutmeg and coconut and stir continuously until the rice is tender and the milk is thick and creamy – the grains of rice should remain separate, not stuck together in lumps.
2. Serve hot or cold, with a little nutmeg grated over the top.

NUTRITIONAL INFORMATION
one serving contains

CALORIES:	305
TOTAL FAT:	13.3G
CARBOHYDRATES:	40.3G
TOTAL SUGAR:	18.8G
FIBRE:	0.1G
SODIUM:	0.3G

Fromage frais hearts
with raspberry sauce

SERVES 4

INGREDIENTS
250 g/9 oz **low-fat fromage frais**

250 g/9 oz **regular fromage frais**

2–3 tablespoons **caster sugar**

RASPBERRY SAUCE

250 g/9 oz **raspberries**, plus extra to garnish

1 tablespoon **caster sugar**

These are such a classic dessert that you can buy ceramic hearts with draining holes in any specialist kitchen shop. You will also need some muslin to line the hearts. Of course you can also use any other pierced containers, such as yoghurt pots – they just won't be heart-shaped. Fill the containers quite full as they will shrink considerably as the liquid drains out.

METHOD

1. You will need to make these at least 2 or 3 hours before you want to eat them. Begin by lining the ceramic hearts with squares of dampened muslin. Place the hearts on a tray or a large plate with a rim.

2. Using a fork, mix all the fromage frais with the sugar. Taste and add a little more sugar if you like. Spoon the mixture into the containers and leave in the refrigerator to drain for at least 2 hours or overnight.

3. For the sauce, blend the raspberries and rub through a sieve. Mix in the sugar and add a little more if you think it needs it.

4. Turn out the fromage frais hearts on to four plates and pour the sauce around them.

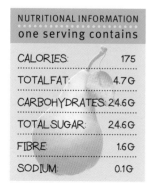

NUTRITIONAL INFORMATION
one serving contains

CALORIES:	175
TOTAL FAT:	4.7 G
CARBOHYDRATES:	24.6 G
TOTAL SUGAR:	24.6 G
FIBRE:	1.6 G
SODIUM:	0.1 G

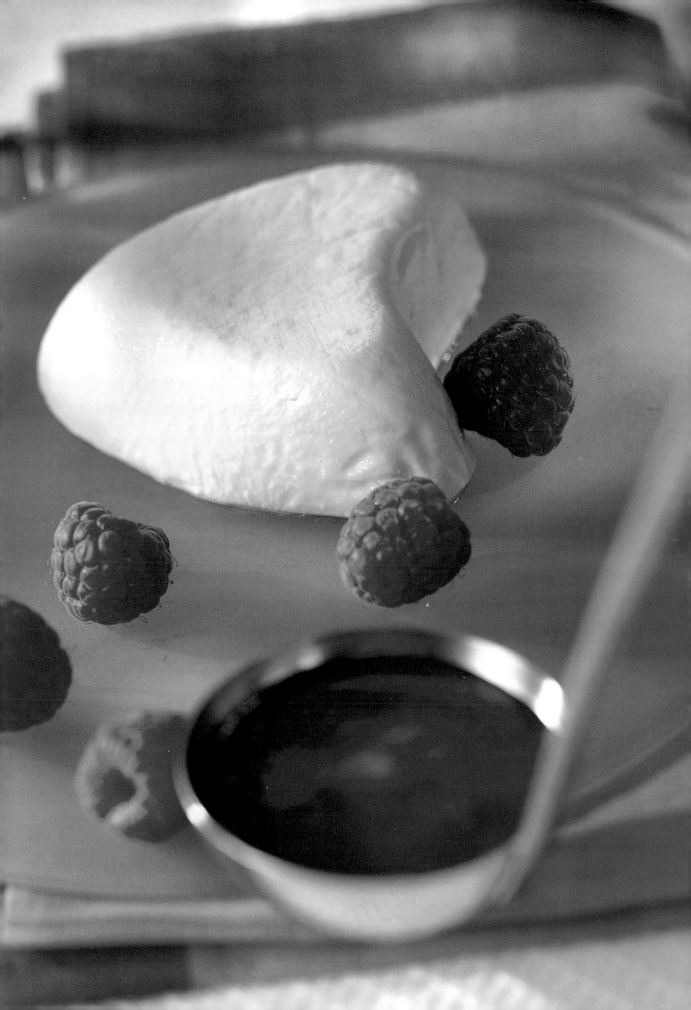

Lemon pudding

SERVES 12

INGREDIENTS

50 g/2 oz unbleached white **flour**

½ teaspoon **baking powder**

325 g/12 oz **caster sugar**

375 ml/12 fl oz **buttermilk** (1% fat)

125 ml/4 fl oz fresh **lemon juice**

2 teaspoons grated **lemon zest**

2 **egg yolks**, lightly beaten

4 **egg whites**

pinch of salt

Buttermilk replaces milk and cream in this recipe and works brilliantly to create a light, mousse-like texture. Cooking it for longer will give you a firmer-textured result.

METHOD

1. Preheat the oven to 180°C/350°F/gas 4. Very lightly spray or brush with oil a 30 x 20 cm/12 x 8 inch ovenproof glass dish and place the dish in a 5 cm/2 inch deep roasting tin. Bring a kettle of water to the boil.

2. Sift the flour and baking powder into a large bowl and mix in just over half the sugar. Add the buttermilk, lemon juice and zest, and the beaten egg yolks, stir to mix and set aside.

3. Whisk the egg whites until soft peaks form, then add the salt and beat until stiff. Beat in the remaining sugar. Gently fold the egg whites into the buttermilk mixture, then spoon into the oiled dish.

4. Pour boiling water into the roasting tin to come halfway up the sides of the dish. Bake for 30-35 minutes, until well risen and golden. (I like it when the bottom layer is quite runny and the top layer just mousse-like. If you prefer, you can bake it for up to 55 minutes for a firmer consistency.) Serve warm or cool.

NUTRITIONAL INFORMATION
one serving contains

CALORIES:	147
TOTAL FAT:	1.1 G
CARBOHYDRATES:	33.4 G
TOTAL SUGAR:	30.2 G
FIBRE:	0.1 G
SODIUM:	0.3 G

Arabic couscous cake

SERVES 12

INGREDIENTS

650 ml/just over 1 pint boiling water

500 g/1 lb 2 oz **couscous**

200 g/7 oz ready-to-eat **dried apricots**,
  chopped

200 g/7 oz moist pitted **dates**, thinly sliced

½ teaspoon ground **cinnamon**

2 teaspoons **lime juice** (optional)

4 teaspoons **orange flower water**

450 g/1 lb clear **honey** (more if needed)

2 teaspoons flaked **almonds**, lightly toasted

TO SERVE

250 g/9 oz thick low-fat **yoghurt**

This can look as exotic as it sounds, but in fact it is not related to any traditional Arabic cake – if anything it looks more like an American Christmas cake, full of glistening fruit. It needs no cooking and can be made in moments.

METHOD

1. Pour the boiling water over the couscous and leave for 8–10 minutes, until the couscous is soft. Leave to cool slightly, then add 150 g/5 oz of apricots, 125 g/4 oz of dates, the cinnamon, lime juice, if using, 2 teaspoons of the orange flower water and 300 g/11 oz of the honey.

2. Line a 22 cm/9 inch square loose-bottomed cake tin with baking parchment. Press the couscous into it firmly, then turn out on to a large plate and peel off the paper.

3. In a small saucepan over a low heat, warm the remaining honey and orange flower water with the remaining apricots and dates. When the fruit is very soft, pour the honey and fruit all over the cake.

4. Sprinkle the toasted flaked almonds over the cake and serve with yoghurt.

NUTRITIONAL INFORMATION
one serving contains

CALORIES:	386
TOTAL FAT:	1.6 G
CARBOHYDRATES:	90.5 G
TOTAL SUGAR:	47.8 G
FIBRE:	1.8 G
SODIUM:	0.1 G

Chocolate angelfood cake
with hot cherry sauce

SERVES 10

INGREDIENTS

100 g/3½ oz **plain flour**

150 g/5 oz **caster sugar**

125 g/4 oz **light muscovado sugar**

12 **egg whites**

½ teaspoon salt

1 teaspoon cream of tartar

2 tablespoons **cocoa powder**

1 tablespoon boiling water

HOT CHERRY SAUCE

750 g/1 lb 10 oz **black cherries**, stoned

2–3 tablespoons **icing sugar**

2 tablespoons **Kirsch**

TO SERVE

150 g/5 oz low-fat **yoghurt**

Here's a light, low-fat cake that's something of an American classic. A word of warning: twelve egg whites whisk up to a huge volume, so you will need a very large bowl, ideally the bowl of an electric mixer. The hot cherry sauce is old-fashioned yet bang up-to-date.

METHOD

1. Preheat the oven to 180°C/350°F/gas 4.
2. Sift the flour and caster sugar together three times and set aside. Patiently sift the muscovado sugar into a separate bowl.
3. In a large bowl, or the bowl of an electric mixer, beat the egg whites, salt and cream of tartar on medium speed, then increase to high speed and beat until stiff peaks form. Gradually beat in the sifted muscovado sugar, a tablespoon or two at a time.
4. Dissolve the cocoa in the boiling water.
5. Using a rubber spatula, gently fold the cocoa mixture into the egg white mixture, then gently fold in the flour and caster sugar.
6. Transfer the mixture to an unoiled loaf tin and bake for 40–45 minutes, or until the top springs back to the touch.
7. Invert the tin but do not remove it. Leave the cake in the tin until cold, about 2 hours.
8. For the sauce, put the cherries, sugar and Kirsch into a saucepan, bring to the boil, then reduce the heat and simmer for 20 minutes, stirring occasionally to prevent sticking. Serve with the sliced angel food cake, together with a tablespoon of yoghurt.

NUTRITIONAL INFORMATION
one serving contains

CALORIES:	236
TOTAL FAT:	1G
CARBOHYDRATES:	53G
TOTAL SUGAR:	44.3G
FIBRE:	1.4G
SODIUM:	0.6G

Roasted plums
with ginger fromage frais

SERVES 6

INGREDIENTS

750 g/1 lb 10 oz **plums**, halved and stoned

3 tablespoons **soft brown sugar**

2 tablespoons **brandy**

4 tablespoons stem **ginger syrup**

4 pieces of stem **ginger**, roughly chopped

150 g/5 oz **fromage frais**

1 small punnet (125 g/4 oz) of **raspberries**

This looks really good made with yellow plums. Crystallized ginger is something I associated with old ladies and Christmas and for years it held absolutely no interest for me. But these things have a way of coming around and I now love it, especially like this, where it spices up the plums beautifully and turns the fromage frais almost into a dessert in its own right. Ginger fromage frais is delicious with all kinds of other fruit and there's no reason why you shouldn't serve it with the apple and pear sorbet (page 152) or the pears in chocolate sauce (page 134) or indeed the chocolate sorbet (page 153).

METHOD

1. Preheat the oven to 200°C/400°F/gas 6.
2. Place the plums on a baking sheet and sprinkle over the sugar, brandy and ginger syrup. Roast for 10 minutes, until the plums have softened and the skins are beginning to split.
3. Mix the chopped ginger with the fromage frais.
4. Serve the plums warm, topped with the raspberries and accompanied by the ginger fromage frais.

NUTRITIONAL INFORMATION
one serving contains

CALORIES:	151
TOTAL FAT:	2 G
CARBOHYDRATES:	29.8 G
TOTAL SUGAR:	29.2 G
FIBRE:	2.5 G
SODIUM:	0.1 G

Brown sugar meringues
with exotic fruit

SERVES 6

INGREDIENTS

6 **egg whites**

325 g/12 oz **golden caster sugar**

1 teaspoon **cornflour**

4 **passion fruit**

100 ml/3½ fl oz **mango juice**

1 ripe **mango**, peeled and thinly sliced

1 ripe **papaya**, peeled, seeds removed, thinly
sliced

Egg white is pure protein so this is a fat-free dessert that looks as elegant and sumptuous as any. Meringues are enjoying something of a revival and brown sugar ones have a lovely flavour. Cook them slowly to achieve a crisp outside and a chewy, marshmallowy centre. They keep for weeks in an airtight jar and can also be frozen. The sharpness of the passion fruit does a brilliant job of cutting through the sweetness.

METHOD

1. Heat the oven to 100°C/200°F/gas ¼ or its lowest setting. Line a baking sheet with baking parchment.
2. Beat the egg whites until stiff. Beating continually, add the sugar a tablespoon at a time, then beat in the cornflour.
3. Using two spoons, form the egg white mixture into 6 large or 24 small meringues, place in the oven and bake until crisp, about 1–1/2 hours. Turn off the oven and open the door, leaving the meringues to cool in the oven.
4. Cut the passion fruit in half, scoop out the pulp and rub through a sieve to extract the juice. Add the mango juice and pour into a sauté pan, together with the mango and papaya. Return the passion fruit seeds to the pan and bring just to the boil, then leave to cool.
5. Spread some of the fruit and juice over each plate, top with meringue(s) and the rest of the fruit. Serve at once.

NUTRITIONAL INFORMATION
one serving contains

CALORIES	281
TOTAL FAT	0.2 G
CARBOHYDRATES	70.1 G
TOTAL SUGAR	66.1 G
FIBRE	3 G
SODIUM	0.2 G

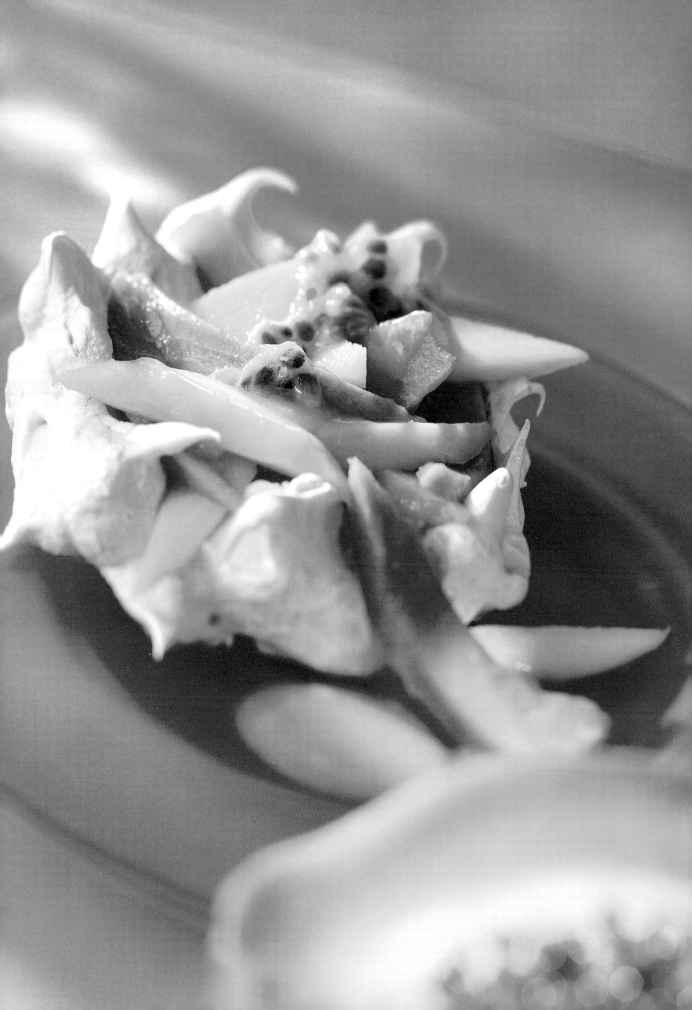

Frozen halva with biscuits

SERVES 6

INGREDIENTS

400 g/14 oz **pistachio halva**, chopped into small pieces

500 g/1 lb 2 oz **bio yoghurt**

1–2 teaspoons **icing sugar** (optional)

BISCUITS À LA CUILLÈRE

1 **egg**, separated

25 g/1 oz **caster sugar**

25 g/1 oz **flour**, sifted

1 teaspoon **grated lemon zest**

1 teaspoon **lemon juice**

25 g/1 oz **icing sugar**

A long, slim biscuit makes an elegant accompaniment to any ice cream or sorbet. This recipe makes about 10 biscuits – any left over can be kept for up to 15 days in an airtight tin. The raspberry sauce (page 142) would also be good here.

METHOD

1. Blend the halva and yoghurt until well mixed, then add sugar to taste and blend until smooth.

2. Transfer to a freezerproof container and freeze for about 1½–2 hours, or until ice crystals begin to form around the edges. Return to the blender and blend briefly, then freeze for a further 1½–2 hours.

3. For the biscuits, preheat the oven to 180°C/350°F/gas 4. Line a baking sheet with baking parchment.

4. Whisk the egg yolk with half the caster sugar until it is thick, very pale and leaves a trail when the whisk is lifted. Add the sifted flour and lemon zest.

5. Whisk the egg white until stiff, then whisk in the remaining caster sugar. Very carefully fold into the yolk mixture, together with the lemon juice, incorporating as much air as possible. Put the mixture into a piping bag and pipe 10 cm/4 inch lengths on to the baking parchment. Sift over the icing sugar, tapping off any excess. Bake for 12–15 minutes, until they are pale golden. Do not open the oven door before 12 minutes, otherwise the biscuits will sink.

6. Leave to cool, then gently ease the biscuits off the paper.

7. Serve the frozen halva with one or two biscuits.

NUTRITIONAL INFORMATION
one serving contains

CALORIES:	524
TOTAL FAT:	23.1 G
CARBOHYDRATES:	55.7 G
TOTAL SUGAR:	51.7 G
FIBRE:	0.1 G
SODIUM:	0.5 G

Mango frozen yoghurt

SERVES 6

INGREDIENTS

1 large or 2 small **mangoes**, peeled, stones removed

2 **passion fruit**

1 tablespoon **caster sugar** (optional)

500 g/1 lb 2 oz low-fat **yoghurt**

Frozen yoghurts are among that special breed of foods that make you feel as if you have had a treat and surprise you by their paucity of calories and their virtual absence of fat. I've kept the sugar level low but you can adjust it to taste.

METHOD

1. Purée the mango flesh with the passion fruit pulp (including the seeds). Taste the purée and add the sugar if you think it needs it. Mix the fruit purée with the yoghurt and freeze for 3-4 hours, or until the mixture is partly frozen.
2. Whisk to break up the ice crystals, then return to the freezer until frozen.

Blueberry frozen yoghurt
SERVES 6

1. Mash 250 g/9 oz blueberries with 3 tablepoons caster sugar and leave to stand for 30 minutes.
2. Purée the blueberries and rub through a sieve, then mix with 500 g/1 lb 2 oz yoghurt and freeze for 3–4 hours, or until the mixture is partly frozen.
3. Whisk to break up the ice crystals, then return to the freezer until frozen.

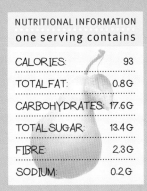

NUTRITIONAL INFORMATION
one serving contains

CALORIES:	93
TOTAL FAT:	0.8 G
CARBOHYDRATES:	17.6 G
TOTAL SUGAR:	13.4 G
FIBRE:	2.3 G
SODIUM:	0.2 G

Apple and pear sorbet

SERVES 6

INGREDIENTS
4 **apples**, peeled, cored and chopped
4 **pears**, peeled, cored and chopped
juice of 1 **lemon**
1 teaspoon ground **cinnamon**
4 tablespoons **caster sugar**

Try adding three or four soft dried apricots to the cooked fruit for a hint of sharpness, a prettier colour and a more rounded taste. Several sorbets of different flavours served in small scoops is a wonderful way to end a meal.

METHOD

1. Put the apples and pears into a large saucepan and add just enough water to cover the base of the pan. Cover the pan and simmer until the fruit is soft, 5–10 minutes. Leave to cool.
2. Blend the fruit to a purée with the lemon juice and cinnamon.
3. Put the sugar into a small saucepan with 4 tablespoons water, bring to the boil and mix with the fruit purée.
4. Transfer to a freezerproof container and freeze for about 3 hours, stirring occasionally.

Blackberry sorbet
SERVES 6

Please do take the trouble to sieve the blackberry purée. It makes such a difference to the final result. A strawberry sorbet can be made in the same way.

1. Sprinkle 100 g/3½ oz caster sugar over 450 g/ 1 lb blackberries and leave to marinate for 1 hour.
2. Purée the mixture and rub through a sieve, then freeze for about 3 hours, stirring occasionally.

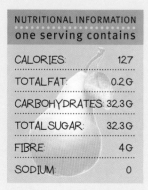

NUTRITIONAL INFORMATION
one serving contains

CALORIES:	127
TOTAL FAT:	0.2 G
CARBOHYDRATES:	32.3 G
TOTAL SUGAR:	32.3 G
FIBRE:	4 G
SODIUM:	0

Chocolate and brandy sorbet

SERVES 6

INGREDIENTS

50 ml/2 fl oz **glucose syrup** (liquid glucose)

100 g/3½ oz **caster sugar**

85 g/3 oz **cocoa powder**

50 g/2 oz dark couverture **chocolate**

2 tablespoons **brandy**

This is based on a Raymond Blanc recipe, to which I've added some brandy. It isn't strictly necessary, but if you're going to indulge, you may as well go the whole hog, strictly within our terms and conditions though. As a committed chocoholic, I think this makes the grade and the only fat comes from the cocoa.

METHOD

1. Put all the ingredients into a saucepan with 50 ml/16 fl oz water and bring to the boil, whisking rapidly. Leave to cool.

2. Pour into a freezerproof container and freeze until crystals begin to form around the edges. Beat until smooth, then return to the freezer.

3. Repeat this process twice more to prevent a granular-textured sorbet. Alternatively, use an ice-cream machine.

NUTRITIONAL INFORMATION
one serving contains

CALORIES	190
TOTAL FAT	5.4 G
CARBOHYDRATES	31.5 G
TOTAL SUGAR	26.1 G
FIBRE	1.9 G
SODIUM	0.4 G

Chocolate mousse cheesecake

SERVES 10

INGREDIENTS

400 g/14 oz dark **chocolate** (at least 50% cocoa
    solids), broken into pieces

375 g/13 oz low-fat **cottage cheese**

300 g/11 oz 98% fat-free **bio yoghurt**

1 tablespoon **icing sugar**

2 **egg yolks**

6 **egg whites**

FOR THE BASE

150 g/5 oz **dried apricots**, soaked in warm
    water

200 g/7 oz **digestive biscuits**

2 tablespoons **brandy**

No, you didn't misread the title: this is made with
fromage frais and low-fat yoghurt. The butter usually used for the base is replaced by apricot purée.
Other fruit purées work as well, for example prune
or mango. It is even better made a day ahead.

METHOD

1. Heat the oven to 160°C/325°F/gas 3. Line a
   22 cm/9 inch loose-bottomed cake tin with
   baking parchment. Melt the chocolate and leave
   to cool slightly.

2. For the base, put the apricots, biscuits and
   brandy into a food processor and blend until
   finely chopped and sticky. Press the biscuit
   mixture evenly over the base of the tin.

3. Put the cottage cheese in a blender and blend
   until smooth. Add the yoghurt, icing sugar and
   melted chocolate and blend briefly, then add the
   egg yolks and blend for a few seconds. Transfer
   to a bowl.

4. Whisk the egg whites until soft peaks form, then
   lightly fold them into the chocolate mixture
   until evenly blended. Pour the chocolate mixture
   over the biscuit base and bake for about 1–1½
   hours, or until just firm to the touch, but still
   mousse-like in texture.

5. Chill thoroughly before eating.

NUTRITIONAL INFORMATION one serving contains	
CALORIES:	404
TOTAL FAT:	17.3 G
CARBOHYDRATES:	50.7 G
TOTAL SUGAR:	39.3 G
FIBRE:	2.6 G
SODIUM:	0.9 G

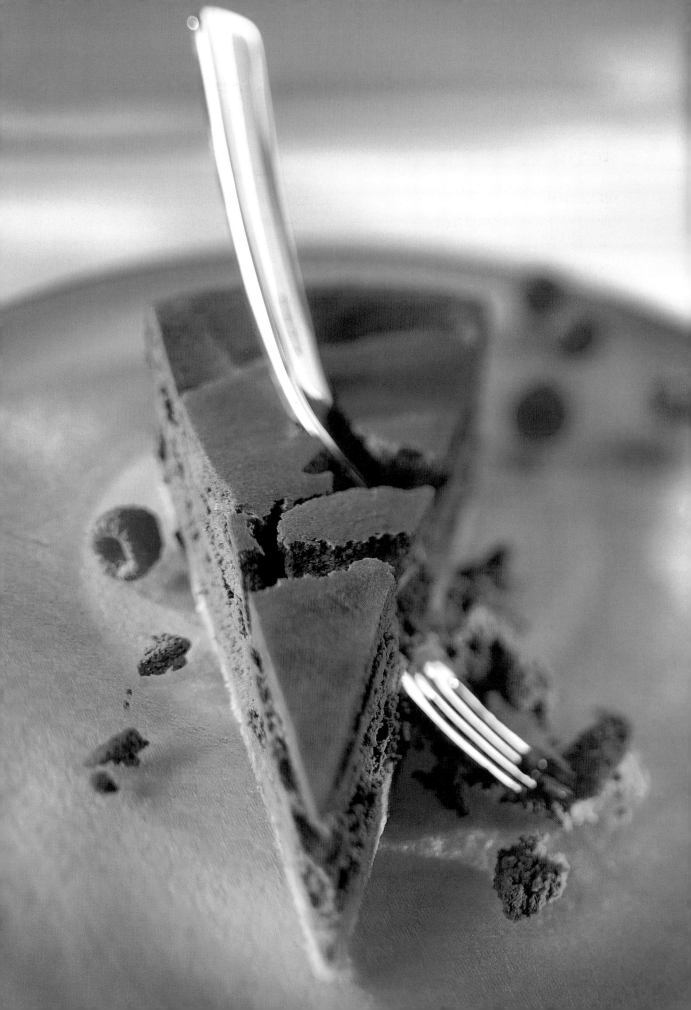

Glossary

Bouillon powder: I sometimes use vegetarian bouillon powder as a seasoning; Marigold brand, sold in health food shops and supermarkets, is made in Switzerland and is gluten-free, with no hydrogenated vegetable fats.

Chocolate: good quality dark chocolate, with at least 50% cocoa solids (preferably 60–70%) is lower in sugar than less expensive chocolate. It is also purer, with fewer additives and no nydrogenated vegetable fats.

Dairy products

I prefer plain, unsweetened, **bio yoghurt**. To keep the fat content low, look on the label to make sure it has less than 2% fat. Bio yoghurt seems to have certain properties that prevent it from separating, which can be a problem when cooking with yoghurt.

Buttermilk, with 1% fat, is a very low-fat product made from skimmed milk and cultured to give it a mild, slightly sour taste.

Fromage frais is the French name for a low-fat soft white fresh cheese. Quark is a German version, and the two are more or less interchangeable.

Smatana is a light sour cream, served with pancakes or the black bean enchilada in this book. Yoghurt could be substituted.

Harissa: a hot chilli paste, served in small quantities with couscous or used as a seasoning. It is sold in tubes or cans in Middle Eastern shops and supermarkets.

Mango juice: the fresh type, sold in cartons, has a more intense flavour. If unobtainable, look for juice with no added sugar or other additives.

Oil: to use a minimal amount of oil for greasing tins or even for sautéing, the cooking spray cans are invaluable. If unobtainable, just brush very lightly with oil.

Sauces: black bean sauce and yellow bean sauce are used to add flavour to some recipes. Look for authentic Chinese brands, but do check the label – a quick glance will show you whether they are full of additives.

Seaweed: the Japanese are the most enthusiastic users of seaweed in cooking. Nori is sold either as flakes or pressed iinto sheets. Look for it in health food shops and Asian stores.

Sun-dried tomatoes: often sold in jars with olive oil and therefore high in fat, these are also sold loose, ready to be rehydrated. Cover with hot water and leave for about 1 hour. Sun-dried tomato purée is sold in jars and tubes.

Tamari: I couldn't do without this Japanese soy sauce, brewed without wheat and therefore gluten-free.

Ume su: Japanese rice-based vinegar made with pickled plums, available from health food shops and Asian stores. The same shops are likely to sell umeboshi plums (pickled in brine) or umeboshi paste.

Index

Alphabetical listing of recipes is in italic